THE
FULL
DIET
COOKBOOK

Crab salad,
page 64.

THE FULL DIET COOKBOOK

DR SAIRA HAMEED

Photography by
Hannah Taylor-Eddington

MICHAEL 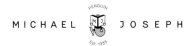 JOSEPH

PENGUIN MICHAEL JOSEPH

UK | USA | Canada | Ireland | Australia
India | New Zealand | South Africa

Penguin Michael Joseph is part of the Penguin Random House group of companies
whose addresses can be found at global.penguinrandomhouse.com

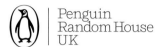

First published 2022
002

Set in TW Cen MT Pro
Colour reproduction by Altaimage Ltd
Printed and bound in Italy by L.E.G.O. S.p.A

The authorized representative in the EEA is Penguin Random House Ireland,
Morrison Chambers, 32 Nassau Street, Dublin D02 YH68

A CIP catalogue record for this book is available from the British Library
ISBN: 978–0–241–62092–2

www.greenpenguin.co.uk

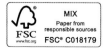

Penguin Random House is committed to a
sustainable future for our business, our readers
and our planet. This book is made from Forest
Stewardship Council® certified paper.

For my brilliant Dad, Dr Khalid Hameed,

who taught me that food cooked with love always tastes good

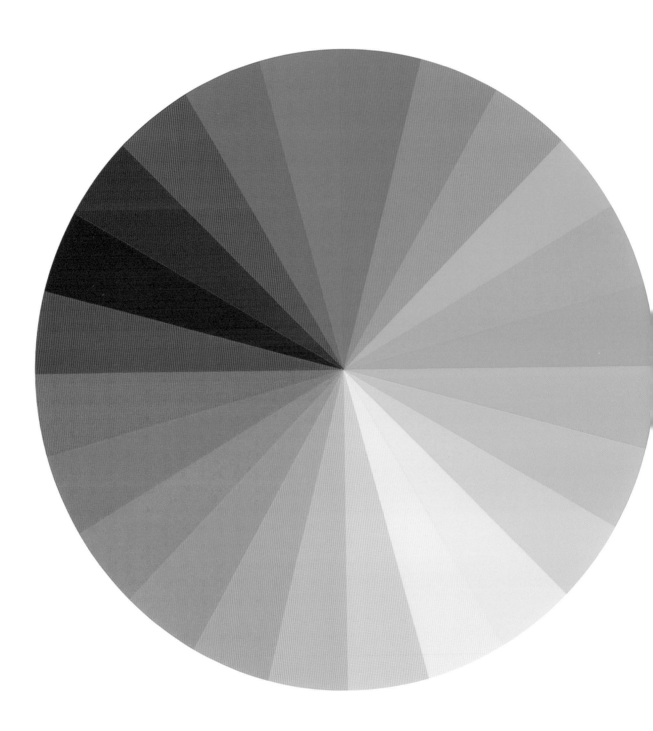

your complete guide to eating on The Full Diet

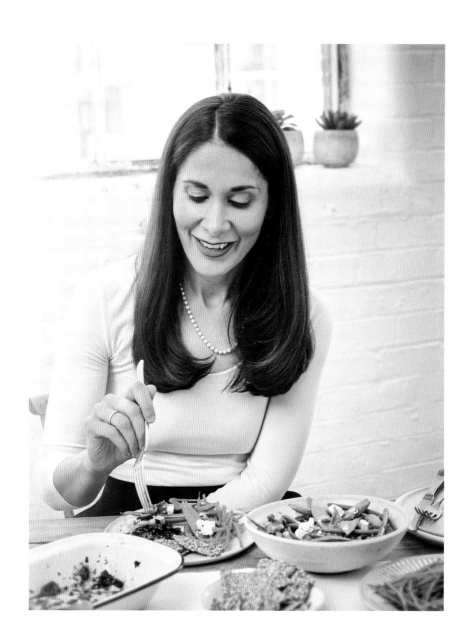

introduction

Welcome to *The Full Diet Cookbook*. I am thrilled that you have chosen this book full of delicious food, science and practical advice, to eat well and feel great. These are recipes cooked and loved by me and my patients over many years, informed and enriched by our own kitchen adventures in cooking delicious food that also happens to help with weight loss as a happy added benefit.

There are over 100 recipes in this book. Each has been carefully crafted to fit with the principles of Full Diet eating, which are summarized in the Programme recap coming up on page 11. But this isn't the full story. My patients have also taught me that our recipes have to be time-conscious, cost-effective, accessible, plant-rich, flexible, joyful and, most importantly of all, deliciously good — and each of these principles is elaborated on in the next few pages.

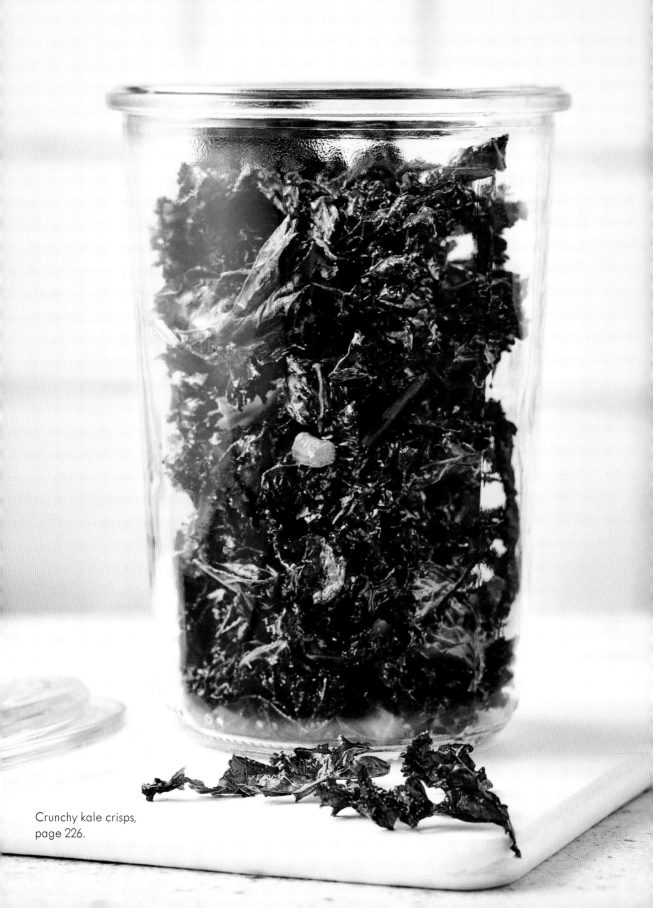

Crunchy kale crisps,
page 226.

The Full Diet

You might be reading this book because you loved *The Full Diet* and are now looking for extra food and recipe inspiration. If so, you can certainly move straight on to looking through the more than 100 recipes and the happy task of planning what to eat. Alternatively, you might find that my summary of the Programme here will be a helpful bit of revision and reinforcement for you.

Or you might be completely new to The Full Diet. If this is you, I hope my drawing together of the foundation principles acts as a valuable guide both to the Programme's eating principles and beyond.

If you have read *The Full Diet*, you'll know that our approach is not about rules and regulations, or being 'allowed' or 'not allowed'. Instead, it is about understanding the underlying science of how your body works and then making a choice about whether to apply that knowledge to your own weight and health situation. This is why each summary point, as in *The Full Diet*, is presented as a choice.

The Full Diet's design is rooted in the scientific evidence base, developed in a partnership between the NHS and Imperial College London, checked through ethical and regulatory approvals and then evaluated in a published clinical research trial. It is now routinely delivered to our NHS patients at the Imperial Weight Centre, one of the country's most highly specialist weight loss clinics. If you look in the back of *The Full Diet* book you'll find over 200 scientific supporting references, the majority of them original, high-impact, peer-review publications in this space. To avoid repetition, I have not included these references again in this book, but please be assured that all the Programme advice I have summarized here is grounded in the same science, and the references are available in *The Full Diet* if you want to find out more about any one particular element.

Food Choices

The food elements of The Full Diet are based on eight key principles. I will cover each in turn. When combined, they form the basis of your Full Diet eating, including the recipes in this book. If you are concerned that there will be a lot to remember or too many changes to take on board, please don't worry. The eight individual food principles combine into more than the sum of their parts, and when taken altogether, you simply end up eating natural, delicious foods, like strawberries, chicken, spinach, full-fat yoghurt and nuts, while steering clear of any foods that were taking your health and preventing you from living at your ideal weight.

How these eight eating principles come together is summarized in the 'Choose to Eat' and 'Choose Not to Eat' food lists in *The Full Diet*, which are also included on pages 242–6 for reference. I always encourage my patients not to focus too much on the foods that were not working for them and which they are choosing not to eat, and to instead celebrate the wealth of taste and flavour available in all the foods that make Full Diet eating such an enjoyable way of life.

Our NHS patients who eat in this way routinely achieve significant, often life-changing weight loss, as well as type 2 diabetes remission, blood pressure reduction, coming off medications, resolution of sleep apnoea, less pain, improved mobility, more energy and a brighter mood. I hope you too achieve these and any other health and wellbeing outcomes that you seek, while at the same time taking pleasure from a life that is full of good eating.

1. Choose to keep your blood sugar levels stable and your insulin level low

When you eat, food is broken down in the gut into its component parts including sugar (glucose), which moves from your gut into your bloodstream. Carbohydrate-rich foods like bread, rice, pasta, potatoes, biscuits, pastries, cakes, sweets and breakfast cereal are broken down by the body into a large amount of glucose, causing the blood sugar level to rise.

On the other hand, foods like eggs, nuts, meat, fish and green vegetables break down into little or no glucose, so eating them keeps the blood sugar level steady.

If you imagine eating a standard (non-Full Diet) 'meal-deal' lunch of a sandwich, a packet of crisps, and a small bottle of orange juice, this can result in the equivalent of 20 teaspoons of sugar ending up in your blood about an hour after eating. For healthy functioning, your body requires just one teaspoon of sugar in the blood at any one time.

This excess sugar in the blood needs to be removed. To do this, your body produces a hormone called insulin, which you can think of as being like a janitor, sweeping the excess sugar out of your blood. Some of the surplus sugar will end up in your liver and your muscles. The rest will be swept by insulin into fat storage and so we gain weight. It's for this reason that, in our patient groups, we call our insulin janitor 'the fat controller'.

What I find so magical about the human body is its resilience. If we choose to eat in a different way, a way that keeps the blood sugar level stable, the opposite process occurs. When blood sugar levels don't rise very much after eating, say, the Caesar salad on page 63 or the prawn fishcakes on page 113, very little insulin is needed to clear sugar from the blood. Insulin levels in your body therefore run low; and low insulin is the signal to body fat to break down. This means that when you eat in The Full Diet way, you give insulin, the fat controller, very little work to do, and so you will lose weight.

2. Choose to eat healthy fats

When cases of heart disease and weight problems started to rise a few decades ago, dietary fat, which had been eaten by humans for millennia, was blamed for these modern diseases. This was a mistake, because it is sugar, rather than fat, that makes us fat. Importantly, in switching to low-fat dieting, what we overlooked was that all fats are not created equal.

Choose to **EAT** fats that nature put on the planet to nourish you	Choose to **AVOID** highly processed oils and artificial trans fats
Olive oil	Highly processed oils, such as corn oil, sunflower oil and palm oil
Butter	Artificial trans fats
Ghee	'Low-fat' cooking sprays
Lard or dripping	Vegetable shortening
Coconut oil	Margarine and other low-fat spreads
Nuts, nut butters and seeds	Ultra-processed fried foods
Full-fat dairy, such as milk, yoghurt and cheese	Shop-bought ultra-processed foods like crisps, biscuits, pastries and cakes
Fats found in natural, one-ingredient foods, such as avocados, oily fish and meat	Any product labelled low-fat, diet or light/lite

Good, natural fats are a cornerstone of a healthy diet, containing essential fatty acids, so called because the human body can't make these fats and must acquire them through the diet for its proper functioning. Many fats, like those found in olive oil and nuts such as walnuts, are also beneficial for cardiovascular health. In contrast, many highly processed fats damage our health and should be avoided, such as artificial trans fats, which are clearly linked to cardiovascular disease.

The Programme is not a high fat diet. Rather, it is about choosing to eat natural, healthy fats such as those found in dairy, meat, oily fish, nuts, seeds and natural oils like olive oil, in regular amounts as called for in conventional recipes within a traditional food culture.

The biochemistry of fats is complicated, but eating should be straightforward. So, for ease of use in everyday cooking and eating, in our patient groups we divide fats into processed or synthetic fats which we steer clear of; and natural fats which we eat and enjoy. Our approach is summarized in the table on page 14, taken from *The Full Diet* book.

3. Choose to boost gut-to-brain fullness signalling

When you haven't eaten for some time, your stomach will send out a hunger hormone message to your brain called ghrelin. You experience this ghrelin message as the sensation of hunger which motivates you to eat something.

When you eat, the gut releases a second message, this time a fullness signal (in the form of the hormones GLP-1, PYY 3-36 and oxyntomodulin). This fullness signal from your gut tells your brain you've had enough, you can stop eating now. There are certain foods that particularly turn up the volume of this gut-to-brain fullness message, in particular protein-rich foods such as eggs, meat, fish, shellfish, nuts, seeds, dairy, tofu and legumes.

The Programme is about eating protein in usual but not unnaturally high quantities, like a 2- or 3-egg omelette (page 52) or a standard portion of veggie chilli (page 178), in order to harness the filling effects of protein without eating it to excess.

This sense of fullness after eating is a revelation for my patients, many of whom joined the Programme after years of feeling hungry on restrictive, low-calorie diets. Instead, by using their Programme food choices to tap into their body's gut-to-brain fullness signals, they now know when they have eaten enough, they feel satisfied and can then easily move on with their day.

4. Choose to eat food, not calories or grams of macronutrients

As you can see, I've summarized the Programme eating advice as:

- Choosing to eat low-sugar foods which keep levels of insulin (the fat controller) running low

- Eating natural healthy fats

- Eating some protein

It's at this point that my patients frequently ask me questions about how much of each of the three macronutrients (macros) – carbohydrate, protein and fat – they should eat. After years of calorie-counting, my patients also ask if I recommend a daily calorie limit.

Here's my response: eating is a pleasure and should be as uncomplicated as possible. When our grandparents or great-grandparents (depending on your age) cooked, they didn't calculate grams of carbs, protein or fat. Rather than eating macros and calories, they simply ate straightforward, single-ingredient foods like chicken, milk and apples. They didn't need a notebook, calculator or app to make their food choices.

The good news is that neither do you.

At its heart, the Programme taps back into this food wisdom by using The Full Diet food lists on pages 242–6 to choose delicious, whole foods. When we do this, the grams of macros and the calories will take care of themselves.

In our published research study of the Programme, we didn't ask our patients to record the amount of carbohydrate or any other macronutrient they ate, and we didn't give them a daily macro or calorie limit. We deliberately took this approach because we have confidence in the body's biology to naturally regulate all of this by simply following the 'Choose to Eat' and 'Choose Not to Eat' lists. I hope that, as my patients find, this comes as a relief, so that you too can liberate yourself from counting calories and macros, and instead just enjoy eating delicious, real food. When you do this your brilliant body will take care of the rest.

5. Choose to steer clear of ultra-processed food (UPF)

The biggest change to our diet over the last fifty years has been the proliferation and normalization of processed and ultra-processed food (UPF), which now makes up 50 per cent of the food eaten in the UK. UPF contains numerous ingredients, new to our diets and which no home cook would use, like emulsifiers, synthetic proteins, flavours, dyes, preservatives and other additives. You'll see these in UPF ingredient lists as odd-sounding substances like anti-foaming agents, hydrolysed protein and E numbers.

UPF is devastating to our health and weight control. Despite food industry messaging that the only issue is 'empty calories', we now know that UPF is unhealthy beyond its high calorie content. UPF generates weak gut-to-brain fullness messages, which makes this food inherently unsatisfying. It is usually low in fibre, high in salt and artificial sweeteners, and often contains poor-quality synthetic fats, like trans fats associated with cardiovascular diseases such as heart attacks. And UPF almost always contains sugar, which hacks the pleasure-generating 'reward centre' in the brain, stimulating a temporary rush or high of the brain chemical dopamine, which keeps us coming back for more.

You will find that one of the great benefits of turning away from UPF is getting back in control of your eating. For many of my patients, recognizing that this food has been designed to hack the brain's biology is a game-changer. This knowledge allows them to stop blaming themselves for a 'lack of willpower' and instead make the choice to turn away from UPF, and the food engineering that was keeping them hooked.

The recipes in this book taste incredible and you will love eating them. But they have been developed in a domestic kitchen, not engineered in a lab. They contain only natural, straightforward ingredients that humans have eaten for generations. These foods will make you feel good but will not hack your brain's biology, so while you will enjoy eating these dishes you will never become addicted to these foods or feel out of control when eating them. This is what eating should be. No chemicals. No tricks. Just taste, pleasure and good health.

My patients lose weight on The Full Diet, but they also report brilliant health outcomes that we hadn't predicted when the Programme was originally designed. From the resolution of skin conditions like rosacea and eczema to the alleviation of daily headaches and acid reflux, their quality of life soars. The research hasn't yet been done to pinpoint the exact mechanism behind these improvements. One theory is that it might be related to an overall reduction in inflammation levels in the body. But I have no doubt that quitting dubious ingredients, like anti-foaming agents, dyes, E numbers and other additives can only have helped.

You can get into the routine of recognizing UPF by checking ingredients. If you come across a dubious-sounding substance, the answers to these three questions will tell you if it is a health-sapping UPF:

- Can I pronounce this ingredient?

- Do I understand what this ingredient is?

- Is this an ingredient that a home cook would have in their kitchen?

If you answer 'no' to any of these questions, then choose to give that food a miss. Be kind to yourself. You deserve better.

6. Choose to avoid artificial sweeteners

A chemical that deserves a special mention is the artificial sweetener. The name says it all: 'artificial'! The Full Diet is about eating real food, and just as we wouldn't want to buy a pot of 'artificial nuts' or a punnet of 'artificial blueberries', the same applies here. Artificial sweeteners stimulate insulin, which works against weight control. The sweet taste will also perpetuate cravings for sweetness, preventing you from recalibrating your tastes to appreciate the inherent natural sweetness of foods like roast lamb, ripened tomatoes, high-summer strawberries and thick double cream.

Coming off artificial sweeteners can be a daunting prospect for many of my patients. But even my patients with the highest pre-Programme consumption of things like diet fizzy drinks and sweetener in tea and coffee do manage it. What I admire so much about them is that mindset shift, recognizing that business as usual – the artificial sweeteners – was not working for them. They weren't at the weight they wanted to be, and so made the brave decision to try something new, which gave them the results they were looking for.

7. Choose to nourish your gut bacteria

One hundred trillion bacteria live in your gut. Everything you eat, your gut bacteria eat too. Fed right, your gut bacteria will help with your weight control, by producing substances which suppress your appetite and extract less energy (calories) from the food you eat.

There is one substance that is particularly important to the health of your gut bacteria – fibre. You can't digest fibre, but your gut bacteria can, converting it into products like short-chain fatty acids, which turn up the fullness dial in your brain's appetite control centre (the hypothalamus).

I ask my patients to eat 30g of fibre a day – the only bit of counting they do (and only initially) to get their eye in. In the Programme, dietary fibre is mostly derived from vegetables but is also found in fruit, nuts, seeds, legumes and pulses.

You can also boost your healthy gut bacteria by consuming probiotic-rich foods that contain a large number of beneficial bacteria. Examples include fermented foods, such as natural or Greek yoghurt, kefir, sauerkraut and miso.

Your gut bacteria also love to eat the phytonutrients found in colourful fruits and vegetables like peppers, carrots, lemons, broccoli and spinach, as well as in tea and coffee, dark chocolate and herbs and spices. In the Programme we call this 'eating a rainbow' – it not only makes your plate look vibrant and joyful but also invigorates your gut bacteria to keep you feeling full and at the weight you want to be.

8. Choose to be cautious with alcohol

Initially, for the first eight weeks of the Programme, I advise my patients not to drink alcohol. Since alcohol is a fermented sugar solution, abstaining stabilizes their blood sugar levels, in keeping with their low-sugar/low-insulin approach. They also avoid the derailing effect that alcohol (or being hung over) can have on food choices. And many note that not drinking for a period of time improves their sleep quality and reduces their stress levels.

Once you are up and running in the Programme, then it's up to you to decide whether to drink alcohol and how much. My advice if you want to drink is to make it worth it, drinking with other people at an occasion that is important to you. Rather than drinking on autopilot, instead choose to drink slowly and mindfully, experiencing all the taste and flavour of the drink – this appreciation will mean you are likely to be satisfied with far less alcohol than you might have expected.

_____

If there is one common tie that binds all of these eight food choices together it's the age-old wisdom of 'Let food be your medicine'. When we choose the right fuel, food is a potent prescription that nurtures mind and body, giving us a feeling of everyday wellness. My patient Stuart, who is four years into the Programme, 3 stone 4 pounds (21kg) lighter and now free of diabetes, sums this up perfectly: 'I choose to look after my body,' he says, 'because it's the only place I have to live.'

The Full Diet:
more *than just food choices*

While your food choices will support you to run low insulin levels, so that you will be in fat-burning mode, there are three other important elements of The Full Diet that also contribute to controlled insulin levels and therefore weight loss.

The first is using an **Eating Window**, a defined period of time when you choose to eat – when your Eating Window is open; and when you choose not to eat – when your Eating Window is closed. It is up to you to define your own timings, based on when you tend to feel hungry, your lifestyle, schedule and preferences. As a benchmark, I advise having an open Eating Window for an 8-hour period.

People vary in the time that they want to open their Eating Window, often choosing somewhere between 11am and 2pm. To avoid any confusion about when the first meal of the day should be, I have deliberately not described any of the recipes as 'breakfast' foods. Instead, you can choose to eat any of the meals in this book when you decide to open your Eating Window and 'break' your 'fast'.

The idea is not to eat as much as possible when your Window is open, but instead to tune in to whether you are hungry and, if you are, to choose to eat something. The majority of my patients find that when their Eating Window is open, they tend to eat two meals and sometimes a snack as well.

When your Eating Window is closed – I advise 16 hours, but see what works best for you – you can continue to drink still or sparkling water, any of the drinks on pages 238–41, fruit or herbal teas, and tea and coffee (with a splash of milk if wanted). When you are deciding on your Eating Window timings, aim to close your Window at least two hours before going to bed.

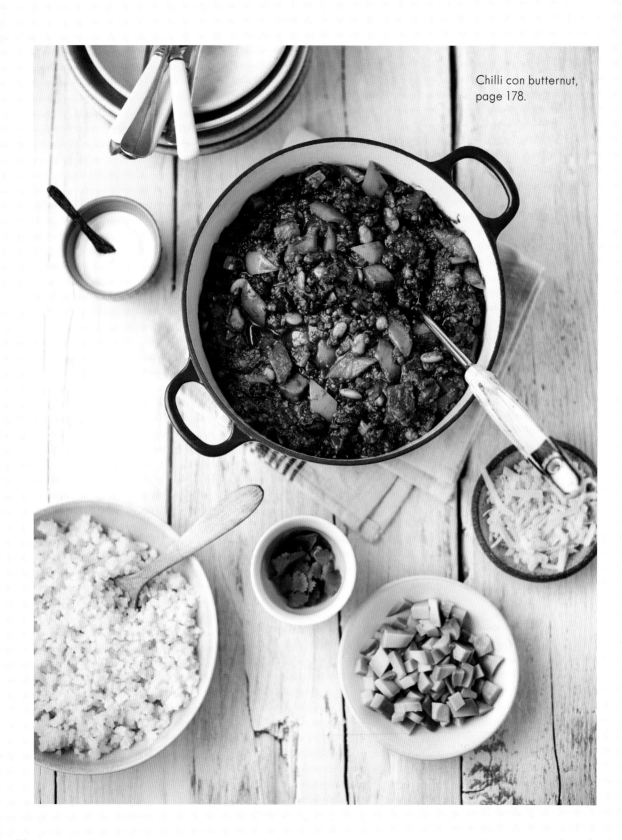

Chilli con butternut,
page 178.

Closing your Eating Window gives you a period of time when there is no incoming food. This keeps your blood sugar levels steady and insulin levels running low. Instead of running on food, your body now gets its energy by tapping into its three fuel tanks – your liver, muscles and body fat.

After a few hours, the fuel stored in your liver and muscles will be used up, and you then tap into your third fuel tank: body fat. The magic of the Eating Window is that when it is closed, this gives you a prolonged period of time of low insulin and therefore plenty of fat-burning, which means even more weight loss.

Exercise and sleep are also fundamental parts of the Programme, because they lower insulin levels through a reduction in insulin resistance, a condition that drives weight gain as well as other illnesses such as type 2 diabetes, high blood pressure and polycystic ovarian syndrome. For this reason alone, sleep and exercise are fundamental to good health, but of course there are a wealth of other health benefits that make both sleep and exercise essential to living a life that feels good.

Exercise makes your body fit and strong and will instil a sense of mental calm too. Many of my patients start to exercise to improve their physical health, but soon see that daily movement is a non-negotiable when it comes to reducing anxiety and lifting their mood, which is why, in the Programme, we describe exercise as our 'mind first aid'.

There is a lot of practical advice in *The Full Diet* on how to introduce daily movement into your life. The key is to view every part of your day, from your commute or school run, to doing the shopping, taking a call or moving between floors, as an opportunity to move and to not be still. 'Make the world your gym' has become a classic Programme mantra. I also advise choosing movement you enjoy, from football to gardening, walking to yoga. If you are having fun, you are far more likely to stick to it long-term.

Sleep is the body's ultimate healer – repairing damage done during the day, filing memories, organizing learning, deep-cleaning the brain and resetting your body's 24-hour time-keeping so that the next day everything happens on time and in the right way.

My patients often ask me how many hours of sleep they should be getting. The answer is that if you wake up feeling refreshed and energized and ready for the day ahead, then you are likely to be getting enough sleep. If you don't feel that way in the morning then, in *The Full Diet*, I advise on strategies to improve your sleep. These include exercising during the day, setting boundaries for evening screen use, carving out 'me time' earlier in the evening, having a 'stop' point for caffeine during the day (12pm or earlier is ideal) and minimizing sound and light in the bedroom. Making these changes takes perseverance, but you will find that if you stick with them, your health will benefit, your mood will improve and you will lose weight – all from the comfort of your own duvet – a true overnight magic fix.

A 'low-insulin way of life'

You can see that The Full Diet uses powerful and diverse elements of the body's biology to reduce levels of insulin, the fat controller. When insulin levels are low, fat is broken down and you lose weight. Aside from weight gain, high insulin levels in the body also drive diseases such as certain cancers, high blood pressure and heart disease. For this reason, in our groups, we also refer to insulin as 'the disease controller'.

By making your Programme food choices, having an Eating Window, moving every day and getting enough sleep, you are not simply on a 'low carb diet'. Instead you are choosing all the mental and physical health benefits, as well as the weight loss advantage, of a 'low-insulin way of life'.

It's not just about the food

One of the reasons that The Full Diet is so effective is that its design has been informed in the NHS by thousands of conversations with our patients, and years of clinical experience in the Imperial Weight Centre of caring for people with weight issues and other health challenges. What our patients have taught us is that weight gain is about so much more than just food.

As specialists in the field, we recognize that weight issues can often be deeply embedded in where a person is right now with their life as well as their overall life story. It is this holistic, whole-person, whole-life, Full Diet approach that is often the game-changer for many of our patients.

If you have read *The Full Diet*, you'll be familiar with the psychology, motivation and behaviour-change strategies that I recommend. I think the best way to summarize The Full Diet mindset is this: 'I'm worth it.'

When you reframe your beliefs, so that instead of labelling your goals as 'impossible' you now view what you want as 'possible', you are tapping into the powerful ability of your brain to rewire itself, creating new habits and behaviours that will bring you the outcomes you seek. When you learn The Full Diet language, so that you are now talking to yourself in a kind and compassionate way, you begin to make friends with yourself. The inner critical voice is replaced by a newfound sense of ease and a quiet inner contentment where it feels good to be you. I hope you will find, as many of my patients have, that this new way of thinking and speaking will also sprinkle in a healthy dose of optimism that permeates life far beyond weight and health goals.

It is from these foundations that self-care becomes a priority, because once you know you are worth it, you will want to look after yourself. From setting a family dinner time that works with your Eating Window, to cooking delicious recipes from this book, all of these actions say, 'My needs matter. I'm worth it.' When you know you are worth it, you will care for yourself with the same nurture and attention that you would show to your children, partner, friends and family.

Developing this Programme mindset has been key to the success of so many of my patients, including Sophia who lost 3 stone 10 pounds (24kg) and came off her blood pressure tablets. Sophia explains things like this, 'The Programme has changed my whole outlook on life. It has taught me to look after and love myself. It has shown me that I don't have to settle for a life of second best — I am worth just as much as everybody else.'

Filling up emotional hunger

None of these recipes talk of 'comfort' food. Yes, we eat delicious and satisfying food which makes us feel physically and mentally well. But we don't eat for comfort because in the Programme we have moved on from managing emotions and soothing ourselves with food. We understand that we have a 'second brain' in the gut full of the same chemical signals, like serotonin, as those found in your 'head brain'. This explains why we experience feelings, including 'emotional hunger' in the tummy, and so we often describe our mood in terms of feeling 'gutted', 'drained' or 'empty'. In the Programme we learn to recognize that this 'gut brain' emptiness is not ghrelin-driven physical hunger, and we develop more effective strategies to 'fill up' that 'second brain' gut emptiness that do not involve 'comfort' food. Instead, exercise, calling a feel-good friend or immersing yourself in a hobby or activity you love will all calm you and make you feel full while, at the same time, putting you in control of your eating, rather than the other way around.

Your goals

You will be more likely to succeed if you keep front and centre in your mind why you are doing this. **What** do you want? **Why** is this important to you? And **how** will you achieve these goals?

In our groups we talk about selecting these choices from a vast online store, 'MyProgrammeGoals.com' and 'placing your order'. You can make sure your order will be fulfilled by visualizing your 'success movie' that you 'watch' throughout the day, 'seeing' yourself buying something you have always wanted to wear or 'hearing' your doctor tell you a medication is no longer needed.

You can also create physical representations of your goals to remind you why you have decided to follow the Programme. Some of my patients set reminder messages on their phone, or stick up Post-it notes or picture reminders. Recently, my patient Kumar, who lost 4 stone 10 pounds (30kg), shared that he uses a photograph of his children as his *Full Diet* bookmark to remind himself why his goal of losing weight and reclaiming his health is so important to him.

This is a cookbook, so, as you would expect, the focus is on food. But I hope this summary reminds you that the Programme is about so much more than eating. The key idea in the Full Diet's holistic approach is that when you believe you are worth it, when you value and look after yourself, weight loss and good health will naturally follow.

The Recipes

The Full Diet recipes are divided into five sections: Eggs, salads and soups; Meat, fish and big veg; Celebration!; Sides; and Essentials and drinks. As with everything in The Full Diet, it is up to you to choose how to use these sections. You might want to make a bit extra so that a side becomes a main meal or choose a Celebration dessert recipe, outside of a special event, for the simple joy of being gathered around the table together on a weekday evening.

I have created a code (page 33) at the start of each recipe to guide your decision-making about what to cook and when, based on prep time, if you're looking for a vegetarian or vegan dish, recipes that are portable, those that are particularly good for batch cooking and dishes that freeze well.

I have also highlighted which foods make a good portable option. We live in a food environment that makes it challenging when out and about to find food that will support your weight and health goals. For this reason, my patients frequently carry their own food, for example taking a packed lunch to work or making a picnic for a long journey or a family outing. What they love about their Full Diet portable food is that it keeps them in control of their eating, avoiding the tricks (and expense) of UPF and Big Food.

You'll notice that none of the sections is linked to eating at any particular time of day, for example 'breakfast', 'lunch' and 'dinner'. This is because people have different preferences about what they like to eat within their own Eating Window timings.

For example, some of my patients prefer to open their Eating Window with a Meat, fish and big veg recipe and then eat something with less involved preparation, perhaps from the Eggs, soups and salads selection later in the day. Others like to open their Window with a quick and delicious dish, choosing to have a meal that requires more cooking in the evening as part of household togetherness and social time. You can of course do whatever suits you best, and it's likely that different days will call for different approaches. There are no rules here, and whichever way that you choose to plan and structure your meals is the right answer.

Mix and match the recipes where you see best, like subbing in cauliflower mash (page 217) to go with your steak in place of piri-piri slaw (page 101) or using feta instead of burrata in your tomato and summer veg salad (page 56) if that's the cheese that you have to hand. As you become increasingly familiar with these recipes, you will find plenty of ways to juggle things around so that the dishes are perfectly right for you. You will also bring to your Full Diet cooking your own know-how and experience. If you think a recipe would taste even better with something added or taken away, then go for it. These are your recipes, for you to cook, to personalize and, most importantly, to enjoy.

Some notes on the recipes

Time

These are recipes for everyday cooks like me and my patients, so the majority assume that you don't have infinite time for food preparation. This is a long-term way of eating, which means that to be sustainable it has to fit in around your work, family and other commitments. While, like me, you might find cooking a pleasure, with plenty of peeling, chopping and stirring sometimes providing a gentle, immersive experience, this book recognizes that a collection of easy, quick and tasty recipes are what's needed for the day-to-day rhythm of your Programme success.

To decide what will suit you best on any particular day, the prep time is indicated at the start of each recipe, importantly also stating the 'hands-off' time where relevant, meaning the dish takes care of itself (roasts, bakes, simmers) while you are getting on with something (or nothing) else.

Cost

There are special occasion recipes in the Celebration! section that do cost a bit more, but with its roots in the NHS, the vast majority of Full Diet recipes have been designed to be budget-conscious and inclusive.

Programme feedback over the years is that, for many of our patients, their pre-Programme way of eating was expensive, including ultra-processed food from the supermarket, meals bought on the go from coffee shops and other outlets, the high price of takeouts and the expense of meal subscription kits.

In comparison, home cooking from scratch, batch cooking when a particular ingredient is on offer and carrying homemade food, for example, taking a packed lunch to work, turn out to be far more do-able cost-wise than many might have imagined. In fact, many of our patients report that they save money with this way of eating, not just on food but on other things too, like more choice of clothes stores to shop at, no fees for diet clubs or weight-loss apps, spending less (or nothing at all) on prescription charges, and fewer (even no) days off work for doctors' visits and hospital appointments.

Accessibility

These recipes don't call for access to long lists of complex or unusual ingredients, but are based around foods that are readily available, no hunting around or specialist shopping required. I have also steered clear of recommending a storecupboard item that is only useful for one recipe, but instead have run a theme through many of the recipes, so that, for example, a spice bought for one dish can be used in several others. I have also recommended only standard kitchen equipment and haven't assumed you have anything more than that – I know I don't!

(Some) Meat

There can be a perception that reducing carbohydrate intake means eating a lot of meat. While meat is certainly part of the Programme, it is just one element of The Full Diet repertoire. For context, in the original *Full Diet* book, just 9 out of the 30 recipes were meat-based. Similarly, while this book gives plenty of meat options, the majority of recipes are meat-free or have a vegetarian option. This approach of including meat as part of an overall way of eating is one that's benefited my patients over many years.

Flexibility

Once you get up and running with your Full Diet cooking, you'll develop lots of know-how for adapting the recipes to make them perfectly right for you. You'll get a feel for how taking something out or adding something in can elevate a recipe to your own classic version, which you pass on to your friends and family when they compliment you on your delicious Programme cooking.

You'll also find recipes in the book that you can pick up and use in another dish. For example, the hollandaise on page 44 is incredibly versatile, working with a huge number of dishes from steamed asparagus to baked salmon and beyond.

See what speaks to you in terms of mix and match, and I hope, as my patients before you have found, that your increasing confidence and creativity bring with them an abundance of pleasure and enjoyment. Importantly, variety is also key. If you love particular recipes, that's the best news I could hear, but I would also encourage you to keep on going, experimenting and trying things out.

The joy of eating

This is a collection of recipes for you but, importantly, this is food for your family and friends too, whether or not they are looking to lose weight. This is why many of the servings are for more than one person. At its heart, Full Diet food is a celebration of delicious, healthy eating, based around fresh, natural foods that your body recognizes as food, so it's a way of eating that everyone can enjoy and benefit from. These recipes are not about you eating in a different way from other people, restricting yourself or missing out. Instead, Full Diet eating fits in with real life, and real life means the shared, sociable and often joyful experience of eating together as a group.

Deliciously good

It's a non-negotiable that every one of these recipes, even if they tick all the other boxes, has to taste great. It's not enough to settle for a dish simply because it has a health advantage. In fact it's the other way around. These recipes are about eating incredible, flavoursome, fresh and exciting food, which just so happens to have the 'side effect' of losing weight and feeling good.

I hope that this collection of recipes brings you as much enjoyment as they have for me and my patients and our families and friends. I hope that cooking these dishes shows you that what you prepare is infinitely more delicious (and often more cost-effective) than the creations of the food industry. Mostly, I hope that your Full Diet recipes reconnect you to what food should be. A delicious and happy experience that also happens to have weight loss, health and wellbeing benefits, in a life that's full of possibilities.

Recipe Category Key

Ready in under 15

Vegetarian option

Vegan

Vegan option

Great portable option

Ideal for batch cooking

Freezes well

eggs, salads and soups

Time and again in our groups, when we discuss the fresh, easy, day-to-day food that my patients are cooking, their dishes fall into one of three categories: eggs, salads and soups.

In my experience, it's these recipes that make The Full Diet so do-able, because this sort of cooking fits into busy everyday life. Many of these meals are either quick assembly pieces, like the vibrant mozzarella, tomato and basil salad (page 55), or require just some basic prep, like building a sausage, egg and spinach stack (page 43) or blitzing a chilled avocado soup (page 76).

But please don't underestimate them – these beautiful dishes are layered with flavours and textures. Despite being simple to prepare, each one can easily hold its own in terms of taste, variety and deliciously good eating, being 'convenient' without any of the 'inconvenience' of ultra-processed food.

Full avo-salsa burrito

Serves 1

Takes 15 minutes

Protein-packed eggs combined with cool guac, salsa and cheese will keep you feeling full. Make extra guacamole if you'd like to eat it as a dip with some vegetable crudités another time.

For the burrito omelette

10g butter

2 eggs, beaten

salt and pepper

For quick guacamole

½ avocado

2 spring onions, finely chopped

juice of ½ lime

¼ teaspoon chilli flakes or chiptotle flakes

For quick salsa

1 ripe tomato, finely chopped

1 tablespoon chopped fresh coriander

a squeeze of lime juice

To serve

20g Cheddar, grated

pow-pow! chilli sauce (page 237, optional)

Make the guacamole by placing all the ingredients in a small bowl and use the back of a fork to crush and bring them together. Make the salsa by mixing together all the ingredients in another small bowl. Keep both to one side until needed.

Heat the butter in a non-stick frying pan on a low heat and swirl round to coat the bottom of the pan. Add the eggs, season with salt and pepper, and stir until the eggs start to set and thicken, then stop and just wait for most of the egg to be cooked (about 2 minutes). Free up the edges with a spatula to help coax the burrito omelette out, then flip over to cook the other side.

Slide the burrito omelette out of the pan on to a plate. Cool for 1 minute. Spread over the guacamole, salsa, Cheddar and pow-pow! chilli sauce (if using).

Roll and enjoy — or wrap in foil for a meal on the go.

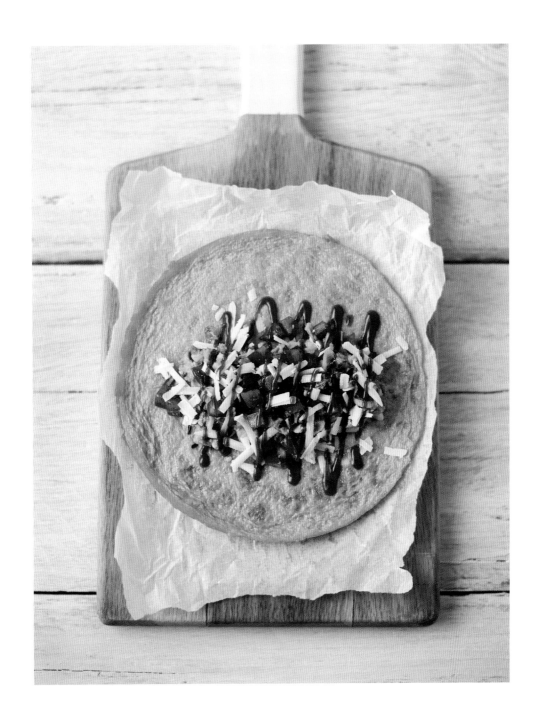

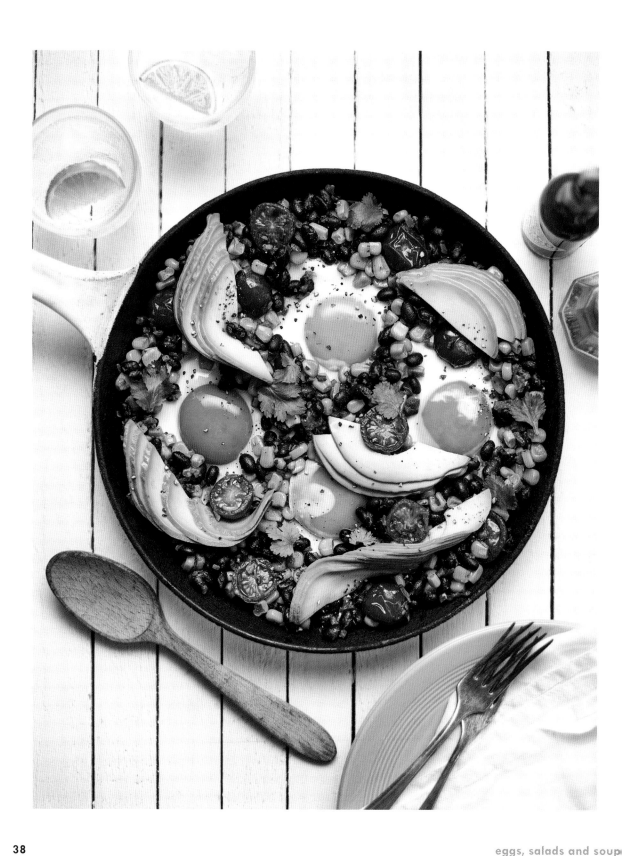

Avocado and black bean baked eggs

Serves 2

Takes 20 minutes

400g tin of black beans, drained and rinsed

1 tablespoon olive oil

1 red onion, diced

8 cherry tomatoes, halved

180g tinned sweetcorn, drained and rinsed (check there is no added sugar)

1 tablespoon chopped fresh coriander

½ teaspoon chilli powder

4 eggs

To serve

1 avocado

coriander leaves

Tabasco Red Pepper Hot Sauce or pow-pow! chilli sauce (page 237)

The baked eggs will dial up your gut to brain fullness signalling, while the avocado is bursting with healthy fats that nourish brain and body. Fibre-rich black beans are a feast for your gut bacteria and – best of all – this dish tastes great!

Tip the black beans into a sieve or colander set over the sink and rinse under a running cold tap until the water drains off clear, which usually takes about 30 seconds. Turn off the tap and allow the beans to drain thoroughly to remove excess water. Set to one side.

Heat the olive oil in a frying pan and add the onion. Cook for a few minutes over a medium high heat, stirring continuously, until softened, then add the tomatoes, black beans and sweetcorn and cook for 5 minutes, until the tomatoes start to break down.

Stir in the coriander and chilli powder, then make four wells in the mixture for the eggs. Crack the eggs in and cook for around 7 minutes, until the whites are set and the yolks are still runny.

Serve with the avocado sliced and fanned on top, with a few fresh coriander leaves and a splash of Tabasco or pow-pow! chilli sauce if you like it a bit more fiery.

Soft-boiled eggs with Parma ham and asparagus soldiers

Serves 2

Takes 15 minutes

Boiled eggs with soldiers just got even better – these crunchy asparagus spears wrapped in salty Parma ham are an exceptionally delicious choice for marching every last drip of eggy goodness from plate to you.

6 slices of Parma ham

12 asparagus spears

15g butter, ideally unsalted as the Parma ham is salty

1 tablespoon olive oil

4 eggs (at room temperature)

salt and black pepper

Cut each slice of Parma ham in half lengthways (easiest with kitchen scissors) and carefully wind each piece of ham around a spear of asparagus.

Heat the butter with the olive oil in a frying pan on a low heat until melted, then add the Parma ham-wrapped asparagus spears. Cook for 2 minutes each of the four sides (for around 6–8 minutes in total), until the ham is golden and the asparagus is al dente (tender but not soft). Season to taste with salt and pepper.

While the asparagus is cooking, place a pan of water on a high heat and bring to the boil. Once boiling, turn the heat down and use a spoon to gently lower the eggs into the water. Cook for 5 minutes for a dippy egg.

Carefully remove the eggs from the hot water, place in egg cups and slice the top off each one. Serve each person 2 eggs, with the Parma ham-wrapped asparagus soldiers alongside for dunking.

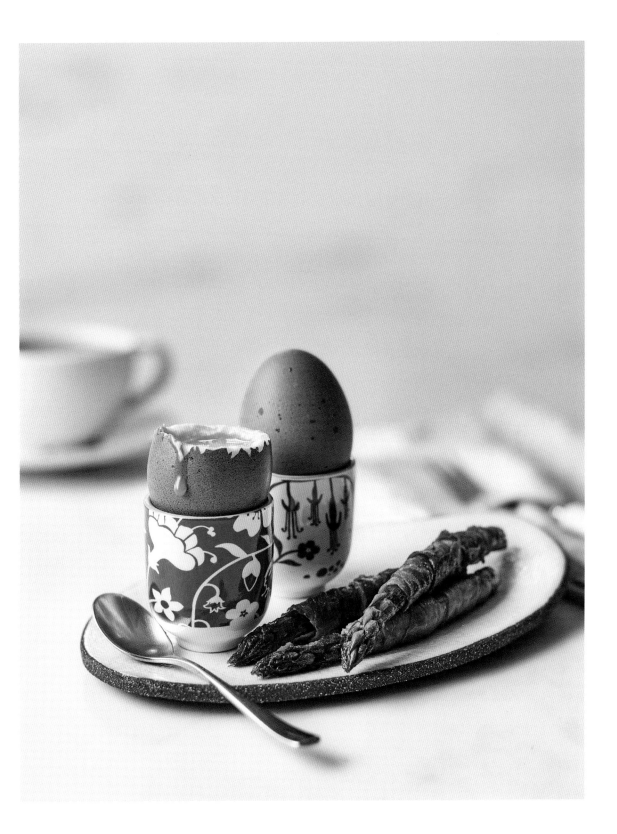

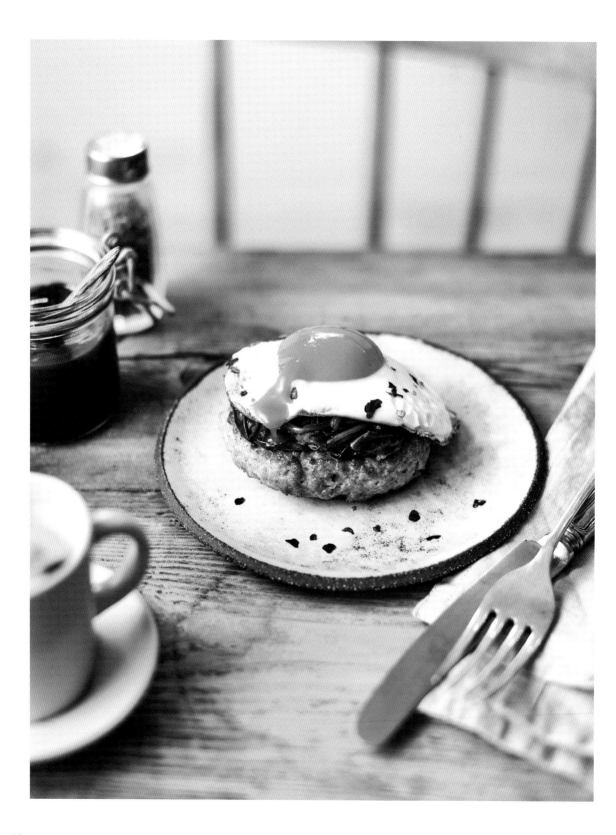

Fully stacked sausage, egg and spinach

Serves 1

Takes 15 minutes

With its meaty, green, eggy goodness this dish really stacks up. Great eaten any time of day, the egg and sausage will make sure your gut is sending out lots of fullness messages while the spinach feeds your gut bacteria plenty of fibre and phyto-nutrients – a quick, easy, delicious all-rounder.

2 pork sausages, very high pork content (more than 90%)

butter (about 2 teaspoons for frying the patty, a bit more might be needed for the spinach and another teaspoon for the egg)

60g spinach

1 egg

a pinch of chilli flakes

salt and black pepper

Remove the sausage meat from the skins by gently squeezing them. Use your hands to shape the sausage meat together into one patty about 1.5cm thick.

Melt 2 teaspoons of butter in a frying pan and add the patty. Cook for around 3–4 minutes each side, until golden brown and cooked all the way through.

Remove from the pan and place on a serving plate.

Add the spinach to the hot pan. There should be enough fat in the pan, but you can always add a little more butter if you need to. Cook until just wilted. This will only take a minute or two on a high heat. Remove the spinach from the pan and place in a sieve set over the sink. Press on the spinach to drain off the excess liquid.

Shape the spinach into a rough round approximately the size of the sausage patty and slide on top.

Pour off any water remaining in the pan from the spinach, add another teaspoon of butter and crack in the egg. Cook for around 3 minutes on a high heat. This will make a really lovely egg that's crispy round the edges. Place the egg on top of the spinach, sprinkle over the chilli flakes and season to taste.

Eggs Florentine

Serves 2

Takes 15 minutes

The hollandaise sauce in this recipe is so easy to make you'll never worry about it curdling into scrambled egg! Hollandaise is also a delicious accompaniment to baked salmon (page 121), steak (page 101), or any other dish you want to eat it with. You can make extra for this very reason, by doubling the hollandaise ingredients, and storing the extra in a sterilized, airtight jar in the fridge for up to 2 days.

For the spinach

10g butter (if using unsalted add a pinch of salt at the same time as the black pepper)

250g spinach leaves

a pinch of ground or freshly grated nutmeg

salt and black pepper, to taste

For the eggs

4 eggs, at room temperature

1 tablespoon white wine vinegar

For the hollandaise sauce

1 egg yolk

¼ lemon, juice only (more to taste)

a pinch of salt

a pinch of ground or freshly grated nutmeg

100g butter

black pepper

Fill a large saucepan with cold water. Cover the saucepan with a lid, place on a high heat and bring to the boil.

While you are waiting for the water to boil, heat a large frying pan and add the butter. Once melted, whoosh the butter round the pan, then add the spinach and season with black pepper. Use a wooden spoon to help keep the spinach moving until it's just wilted. Turn the heat off, pour any excess liquid out of the pan, then season with salt, pepper and nutmeg, and keep the spinach to one side.

Next, make the hollandaise sauce. Put the egg yolk, lemon juice, salt, nutmeg and some black pepper into a mini blender. Melt the butter over a medium heat until it starts to bubble. Remove from the heat and start the motor running on the mini blender. Slowly drizzle in the hot butter. Check the seasoning, add more lemon juice if needed, and once you are happy, it's time to poach the eggs.

Crack the eggs into 4 ramekins or small cups.

Add the vinegar to the boiling water, then turn the heat right down to a simmer. One by one, carefully tip the eggs out of the ramekins into the water to poach. Cook for 3 minutes, then gently remove with a slotted spoon and drain on kitchen paper.

Divide the spinach between two plates, and top each pile with 2 poached eggs and some of the hollandaise. Add a final twist of black pepper to serve.

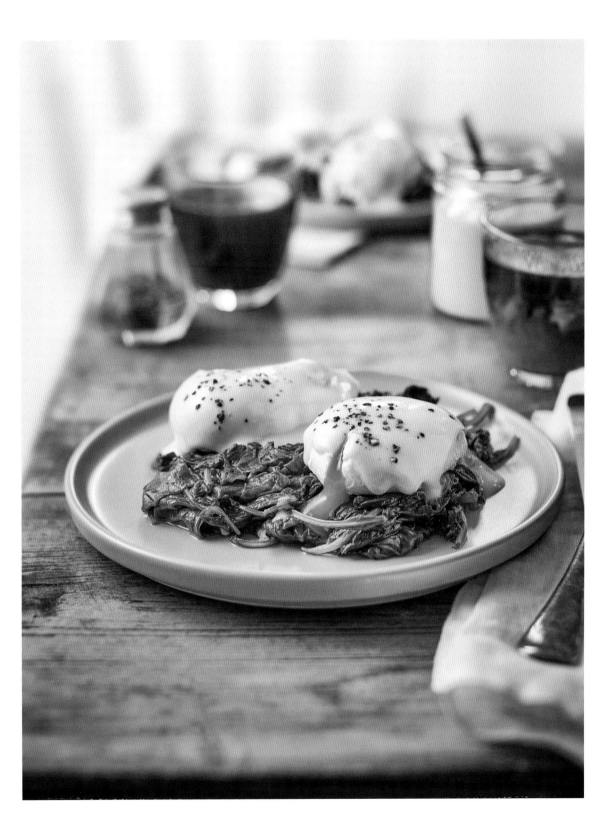

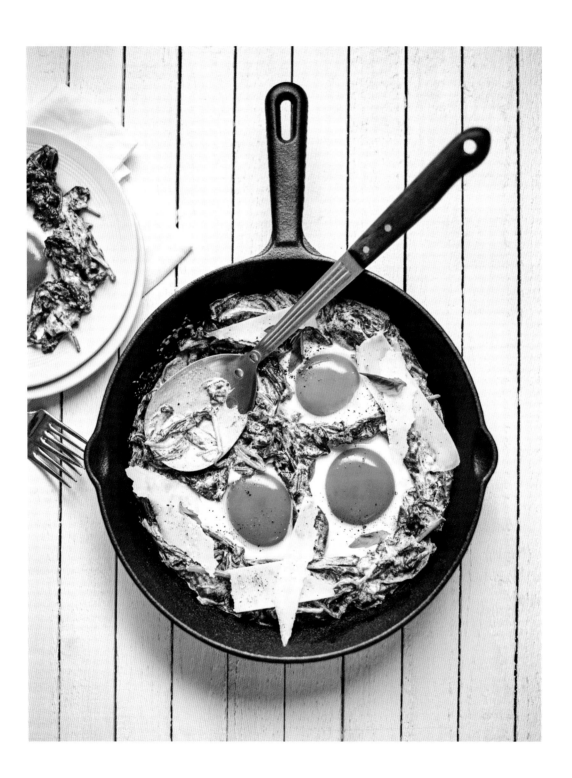

Green Eggs

(if vegetarian
Parmesan used)

Serves 2

Takes 20 minutes

2 tablespoons olive oil

240g spinach leaves

2 tablespoons basil pesto
 (page 85, or if shop-
 bought, check there are no
 dubious ingredients)

2 tablespoons crème fraîche
 (or double cream)

4 eggs

salt and black pepper

To serve (all optional)

fresh basil leaves

Parmesan shavings

pow-pow! chilli sauce
 (page 237) or dried
 chilli flakes

A simple and super delicious one-pan wonder – the mineral rich spinach cuts through the velvet crème fraîche, all combining with the pesto to bathe the eggs in gorgeous green goodness.

Heat a large frying pan on a medium high heat and add the oil. Add the spinach, season and, keeping the spinach moving with a wooden spoon, cook until most of the leaves have wilted.

Once most of the spinach has wilted, add the basil pesto and crème fraîche. Stir to combine, then make four wells in the mix.

Crack 1 egg into each well and cook for around 7 minutes, until the whites are set and the yolks are runny. If you have too much mix under the eggs, they can take a bit longer – popping a lid on the pan will help speed up the cooking.

To serve, divide the spinach and eggs between two plates, add some fresh basil, Parmesan shavings and – if you want an extra hot kick – a dash of pow-pow! chilli sauce or a sprinkle of dried chilli flakes.

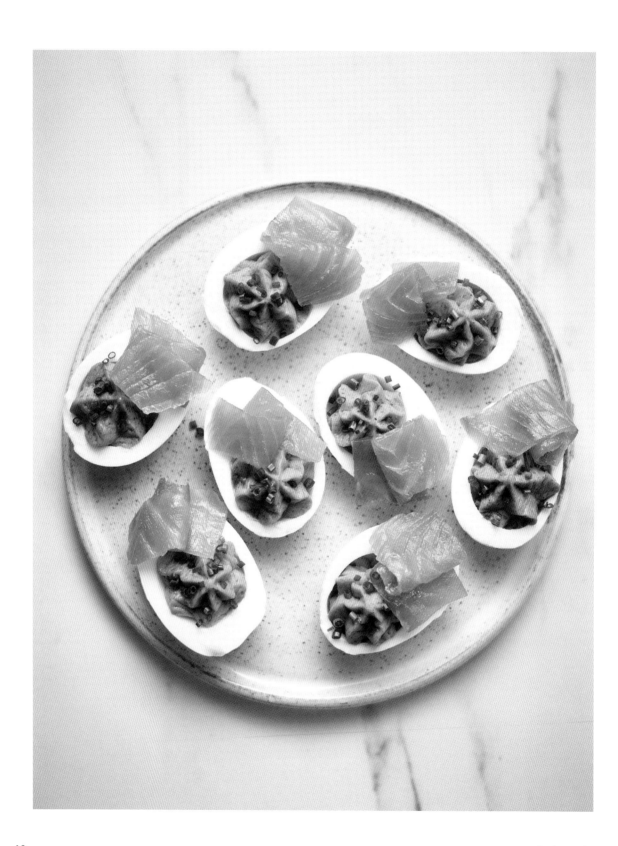

Smoked salmon devilled eggs

Serves 2

Takes 20 minutes,
plus cooling time

4 eggs (at room temperature)

2 tablespoons mayonnaise
(homemade (page 234)
or shop-bought)

2 teaspoons olive oil

1 teaspoon English mustard

¼ teaspoon hot smoked
paprika

a pinch of salt

To serve

40g smoked salmon slices or
trimmings

1 teaspoon chopped chives
or, if not available, parsley
or coriander also work well

black pepper

It's said that the 'devil is in the detail' – when it comes to these eggs, the devilish detail is the kick of the paprika and the mustardy yolks, gloriously nestled in the egg white halves and topped with smoked salmon – devilishly delicious!

Bring a pan of water to the boil, then carefully add the eggs and cook for 8 minutes. Remove from the heat, place the pan in the sink and run cold water over the eggs, before leaving them to fully cool.

Peel the eggs, then slice them in half lengthways and pop out the yolks into a small mixing bowl. Use a fork to help start breaking up the yolks, then add the mayonnaise, olive oil, mustard, paprika and salt. Mix well to combine.

Spoon teaspoons of the mix back into the egg white halves, or, if you are serving to guests, for some extra wow, you can pipe the mix in. Tear the salmon into small pieces and place on top of the egg yolk mix. Scatter over some chives (or an alternative like chopped parsley or coriander) and finally add a twist of black pepper.

This would be delicious with a simple green salad. You can also serve any smoked salmon that's left over in the packet on the side if you like.

Red, amber, green frittata

Serves 6

Takes 25 minutes

40g butter

1 tablespoon olive oil

1 onion, finely diced

1 bunch of asparagus, cut into 1cm pieces (or ½ head of broccoli, or 100g peas)

100g ham, cut into 1cm pieces

10 eggs, beaten

150g Cheddar, grated

1 teaspoon chilli flakes

salt and black pepper

To serve

big handfuls of rocket, watercress and spinach salad leaves

squeeze of lemon or lime juice

drizzle of olive oil

pinch of salt

Delicious piping hot from the oven, melted golden Cheddar bubbling alongside the ham's pink meatiness, shot through with the fresh green goodness of asparagus spears, all lifted by a chilli kick. Alternatively, just as good served cold for packed lunches and picnics.

Preheat the oven to 190°C/170°C fan/gas 5.

Heat the butter and oil in a 25cm non-stick oven-safe frying pan on a medium heat and add the onion and asparagus (or broccoli or peas if using instead). Cook for 8–10 minutes, stirring occasionally, until softened and starting to caramelize.

Reduce the heat a little and add the ham, eggs, Cheddar, chilli flakes and a little seasoning, carefully stirring to combine. Keep stirring for just another minute or two until the egg begins to thicken.

Transfer the whole pan to the oven and cook for 12–15 minutes, until the frittata has risen slightly, the middle doesn't wobble when you gently shake the pan and it is a lovely golden brown.

Remove from the oven and allow to cool slightly in the pan. Run a spatula around the edge of the pan and slightly underneath the frittata, giving the pan a little shake to help coax out the frittata, then slide it out on to a chopping board or large serving plate. Next plate up big handfuls of salad leaves and dress with a squeeze of fresh lemon or lime juice, a drizzle of olive oil and a pinch of salt. Serve the frittata on top of or alongside the salad leaves.

Cut into 6 slices and either eat straight away or allow to cool, then store in the fridge in an airtight container for another time or for a delicious portable meal on the go. If storing, keep without the salad and add the leaves fresh when serving.

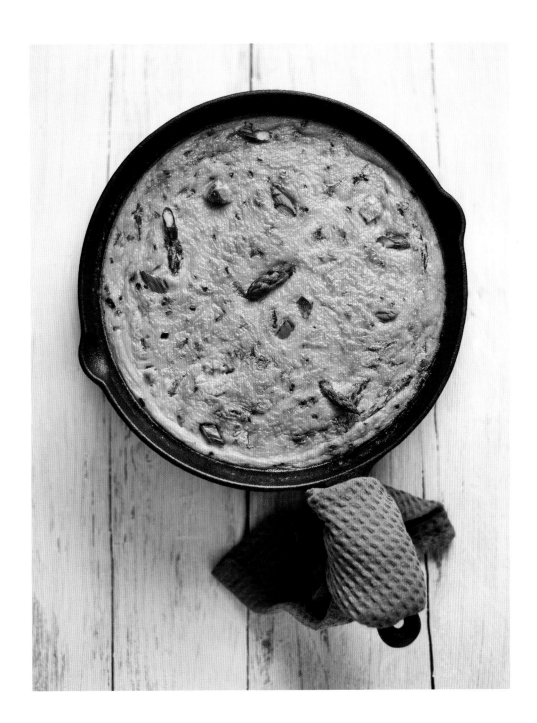

Omelette

Serves 1

Takes 5–10 minutes

Base recipe

2 or 3 eggs

salt and black pepper

a knob of butter, for frying

Filling ideas

20g Cheddar, grated

20g ham, diced

1 tablespoon frozen peas

¼ teaspoon chilli flakes

OR

20g Cheddar, grated

20g kimchi, roughly chopped

1 teaspoon chopped chives

OR

30g roasted peppers, deseeded and diced

20g feta, crumbled

½ teaspoon chipotle chilli flakes

To serve (all optional)

avocado

cherry tomatoes

If omelettes are a daunting prospect because of the flip then there is no need to worry – this no-flip method works every time. And if omelettes are already part of your repertoire, read on because this recipe will give you even more ideas for this versatile culinary classic – the filling protein goodness of the eggs permeated with sweet golden butter is the ideal base for a wealth of additions and flavours. Take inspiration from these possibilities, mix and match, and create your own version of this timeless go-to.

Crack the eggs into a jug and beat well with a fork or a small whisk. Add a little seasoning and beat again.

Heat a non-stick, ovenproof frying pan on a low heat and add the knob of butter. Shake the pan to coat the whole base, then add the beaten egg. Make sure all the base of the pan is covered by the egg, then cook very slowly.

While the egg is cooking, preheat the grill to a medium setting.

Use a spatula or a wooden spoon to stir the egg and move it all around until it just starts to set, then sprinkle over whichever fillings you are using and place the pan under the grill to cook the filling and the top of the omelette.

Once the filling is cooked and the top of the omelette is set, remove from the grill, slide the omelette on to your plate and enjoy.

For some extra depth of texture and flavour, if you'd like to, serve with avocado slices and cherry tomatoes.

Fully loaded avocados

  Vegan

Serves 1

Takes 5 minutes

1 avocado, halved

100g hummus

25g feta, crumbled (leave out for a vegan option or substitute with a vegan cheese alternative)

6 cherry tomatoes, quartered

6 olives, halved

2 teaspoons mixed seeds (including sunflower seeds, poppy seeds, pumpkin seeds)

1 teaspoon extra virgin olive oil

black pepper

As a simple assembly job, this takes less time than heating up a ready meal. The creamy, healthy fat of the avocado is offset by the goodness of the hummus and the tart saltiness of the feta and olives, all topped off with a sweet crunch from the tomatoes and seeds. Loaded is the word! Ideal to eat at home or carried as a packed lunch.

Take the avocado and place the halves on your plate or in your lunchbox.

Fill the holes left by removing the stone with the hummus. Crumble over the feta, then add the cherry tomatoes, olives and lastly the seeds.

Add a drizzle of extra virgin olive oil and a twist of black pepper. Serve with your choice of green veg if wanted.

If you are taking this in a lunchbox, you may want to remove the avocado from its skin first and rub with lemon juice to prevent browning.

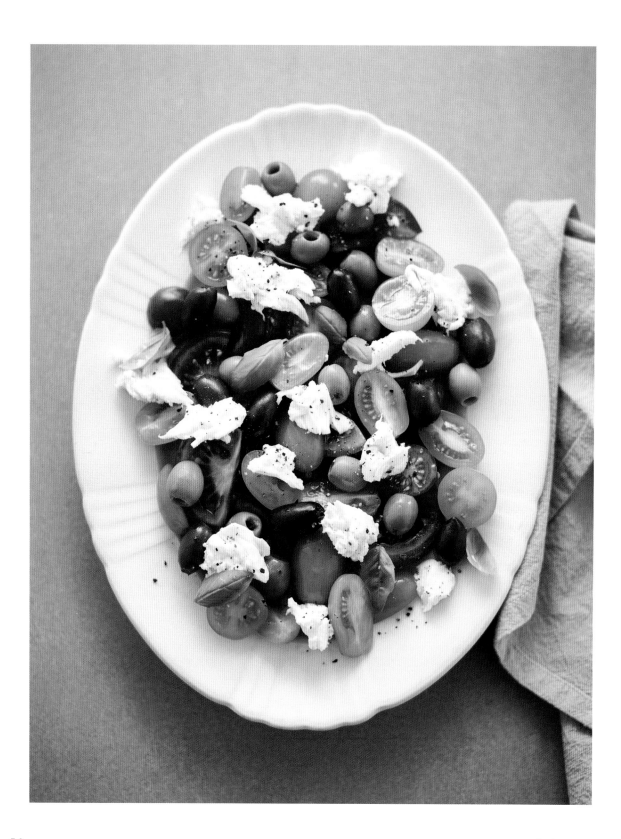

Mozzarella, tomato and basil salad

Serves 2

Takes 10 minutes

300g mixed variety tomatoes, sliced

1 small sweet onion, thinly sliced into rounds (optional, depending on whether you like raw onion)

200g buffalo mozzarella, drained and roughly torn

40g pitted olives (mixed or green or black)

10 basil leaves

For the dressing

2 tablespoons extra virgin olive oil

1 tablespoon white wine vinegar

salt and black pepper

More of an assembly piece than a recipe, this colourful dish takes just minutes to put together but tastes so much more than the sum of its parts. Take the mozzarella out of the fridge about an hour before using – allowing it to come up to room temperature, which opens up the tangy creaminess of the cheese. You can also substitute the mozzarella with burrata if available. Tomatoes are best stored out of the fridge, which prevents the sweet flavour from seizing up when fridge cold. Enjoy as a main or a side – also ideal as part of a spread at a party, barbecue or picnic.

Take a large serving plate and lay out the slices of tomato. Use a variety of sizes and colours (you don't have to be neat, often a random arrangement looks prettier). Top with the onion slices (if using), mozzarella, olives and basil leaves.

To make the dressing, shake the oil and vinegar together in a clean jam jar along with some salt and pepper, and drizzle over the salad.

Check for seasoning and serve at room temperature.

Burrata with tomato and summer veg salad

Serves 2

Takes 15 minutes

200g burrata or alternatively mozzarella will also work well

40g rocket

1 courgette, peeled into ribbons

300g mixed ripe tomatoes, sliced

4 asparagus stalks, ends trimmed, shaved into ribbons using a vegetable peeler

4 radishes, thinly sliced

20 basil leaves

2 tablespoons extra virgin olive oil

salt and black pepper

1 unwaxed lemon, zest and juice (to taste) (optional)

There is a certain joy in cutting into the ivory burrata dome and watching its silky cream rushing out on to the rainbow of sweet, crunchy vegetables. Ideal as a meal or a side at a picnic, lunch party or barbecue, this salad is a taste of fresh summer goodness.

For a really creamy, oozing burrata, take the cheese out of the fridge 1–2 hours before using, keeping the cheese covered with either kitchen paper or a bowl.

Take a large serving plate and lay down the rocket as your base. Start to layer up your salad, adding the courgette, tomatoes, asparagus and radishes.

Place the burrata in the middle, add the basil leaves, then drizzle over the extra virgin oil and add some seasoning.

The juices of the tomatoes and the creamy centre of the burrata usually mean you don't need anything else, but you could always add a squeeze of lemon juice and a sprinkling of lemon zest if you'd like that extra citrus freshness.

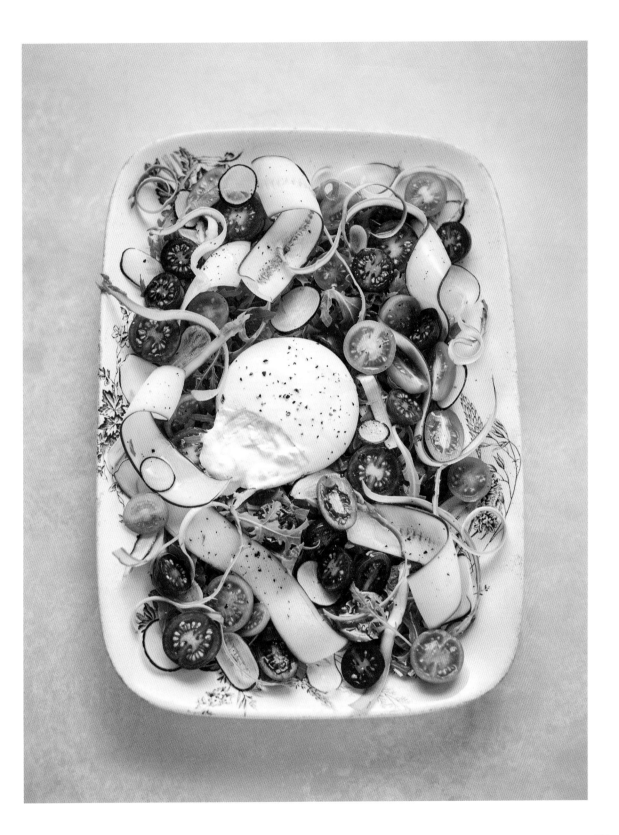

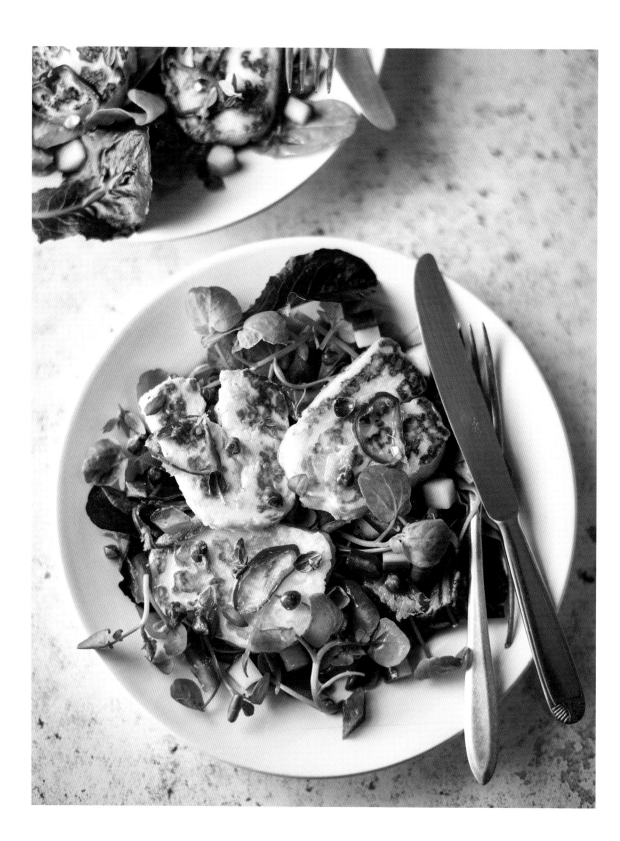

Halloumi and caper salad

Serves 2

Takes 15 minutes

A salad of soft green leaves, topped with the searing, salty goodness of the hot halloumi, perfectly balanced by the acidity of the capers and lemon. There is also something incredibly pleasing in inadvertently creating the dressing as you go along!

3 tablespoons olive oil

250g halloumi, cut into 6 slices

1 red chilli, sliced (leave the seeds in if you like the heat)

2 tablespoons capers, drained and rinsed

1 unwaxed lemon, zest and juice (to taste)

To serve

50g soft green salad leaves, such as spinach, butter lettuce or lamb's lettuce

3 ripe tomatoes, chopped

¼ cucumber, chopped

1 teaspoon lemon thyme leaves or alternatively 1 teaspoon of fresh thyme or oregano

black pepper

Heat the olive oil in a large frying pan on a medium heat and add the halloumi. Cook for 2–3 minutes, until golden brown, then turn the slices over and cook for another 2–3 minutes on the other side.

Add the chilli and capers to the pan, followed by the lemon zest and juice. Shake the pan to blend everything together, then remove from the heat and set to one side.

Divide the leaves, tomatoes and cucumber between your serving plates. Top with 3 slices each of the halloumi and divide the capers. Sprinkle over the thyme leaves and a little black pepper. It's unlikely you'll need salt, as the capers and halloumi are naturally salty. Pour over the juices from the pan as the dressing and serve immediately.

The full house salad

Serves 2

Takes 20 minutes

Bursting with colourful goodness for your gut bacteria, healthy fats and protein that keeps you satisfied with a burst of fullness hormone – this is a full house of a salad. Perfect for eating at home or as a portable meal on the go.

For the chicken

4 chicken thighs, skinless and boneless (you can choose not to include chicken if you would like this to be a vegetarian salad)

1 teaspoon olive oil

1 teaspoon dried mixed herbs

salt and black pepper

For the salad

2 eggs, hard-boiled and diced

1 avocado, diced

2 tomatoes, diced

½ cucumber, diced

1 romaine lettuce, chopped

200g tinned sweetcorn (with no added sugar), drained

For the dressing

2 tablespoons full-fat Greek yoghurt

1 tablespoon olive oil

½ lemon, juice only

2 teaspoons dried oregano

½ teaspoon of additional spice flavour like paprika, or cumin or coriander, depending on your taste preference

salt and black pepper

To serve

roughly chopped fresh herbs, such as parsley or chives

super seeded crackers, crumbled (page 230) (optional)

If using chicken, preheat your grill to a medium high setting and line a shallow roasting tin with foil.

Place the chicken thighs in the tray, then drizzle over the olive oil, season with salt and pepper and add the mixed herbs. Toss to coat, then place under the hot grill. Cook for 4–6 minutes each side (or until cooked through).

Once the chicken is cooked, remove from the heat and place on a chopping board. Leave to rest until cool enough to pick up in your hands, then cut into chunks and place in a bowl or lunchbox.

Next add the diced egg – which has been hard-boiled in boiling water for 8 minutes – the avocado, tomatoes, cucumber, lettuce and sweetcorn. Mix well to combine.

For the dressing, put all the ingredients into a small bowl and whisk well to combine (or use a clean jam jar and shake well), then drizzle over the chopped salad and toss to coat.

Finally, add the chopped fresh herbs and, if you like a little crunch, some crumbled super seeded crackers.

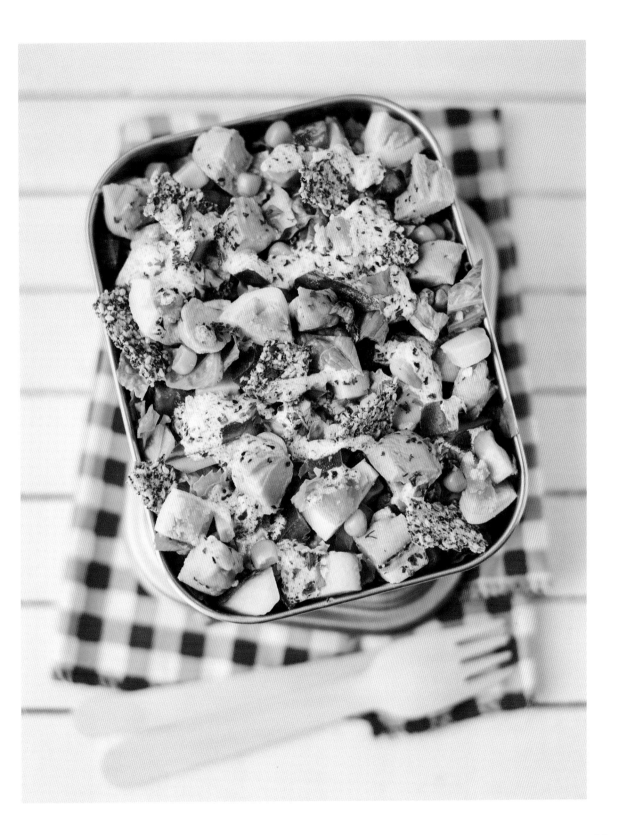

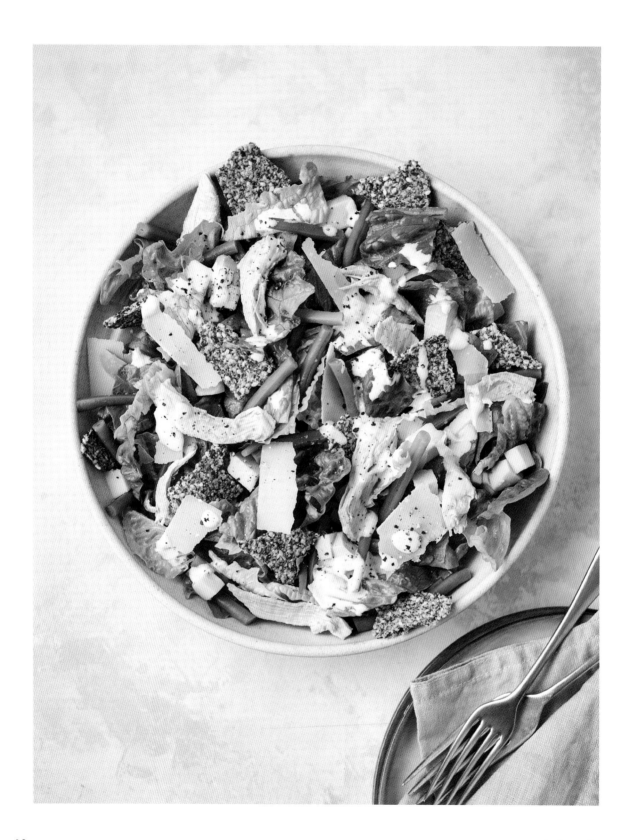

The full Caesar

(if vegetarian Parmesan used)

Serves 2

Takes 15 minutes

There are few things better than the marriage of crisp, fresh lettuce leaves with the salty richness of Caesar dressing. You can improvise on this recipe, using it as a base and adding whatever you happen to have in the fridge. I often add a couple of hard-boiled eggs or some crispy bacon rashers, as well as any leftovers I might have like green beans or roast chicken.

For the salad

1 head of romaine lettuce, cut into chunks

100g green beans, steamed and cut into thirds, or raw sugarsnaps (both optional)

1 avocado, cut into chunks

200g leftover roast chicken (optional)

10 anchovies (optional)

For the dressing

3 tablespoons mayonnaise (homemade (page 234) or shop-bought)

2 tablespoons full-fat Greek yoghurt

½ lemon, juice only

1 small clove of garlic, sliced

2 anchovies (optional)

2 tablespoons grated Parmesan

black pepper

To serve

super seeded crackers, crumbled (page 230)

Parmesan shavings

To make the dressing, place all the ingredients in a mini chopper and blitz until smooth. Check the seasoning and balance the salt, lemon and Parmesan until you are happy.

Place all the salad ingredients in a large mixing bowl and add the dressing. Toss to coat the leaves in the dressing, then divide between two serving plates.

Top with crumbled super seeded cracker croutons and Parmesan shavings.

Crab salad

Serves 1

Takes 15 minutes

30g soft-leaved lettuce, such as little gem, butter lettuce, batavia or escarole

10g rocket

4 asparagus spears, shaved thinly into ribbons using a vegetable peeler

3 radishes, thinly sliced

½ avocado, peeled and thinly sliced

150g white crab meat (fresh or tinned)

For the dressing

1 heaped tablespoon mayonnaise (homemade (page 234) or shop-bought)

½ lemon or lime, juice only

1 teaspoon finely chopped fresh tarragon

1 red chilli, deseeded (or leave the seeds in if you like the heat) and finely chopped

salt and black pepper

To serve

chopped chives (optional)

Salty crab meat nestled in a crunchy, colourful salad, elevated by the fiery chilli dressing is a delicious taste of the seaside, wherever you are. Eat at home, or perfect carried as on-the-go food.

Mix the dressing ingredients in a small bowl or shake together in a clean jam jar, and keep to one side.

Place the salad leaves in a serving bowl or lunchbox, and top with the asparagus, radishes and avocado.

Scatter over the crab meat, then pour over the dressing and toss to combine.

Garnish with chopped chives if using.

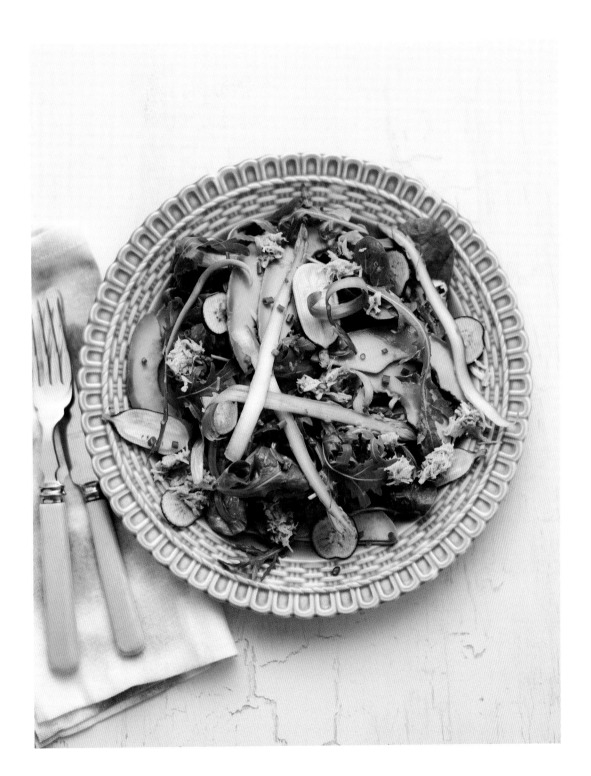

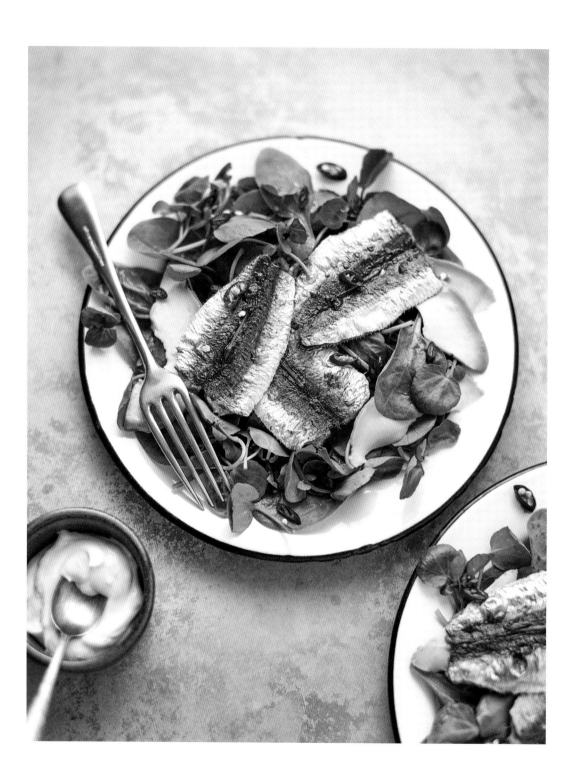

eggs, salads and soup

Sardine, avocado and watercress salad

Serves 2

Takes 15 minutes

The peppery, heady watercress is a perfect foil to the creamy avocado and briny sardines. Serve with lemony mayonnaise for that extra layer of velvety citrus zing.

For the sardines

20g butter

6 sardines, butterflied, or 135g tin of sardines in extra virgin olive oil, drained

For the salad

80g watercress

40g spinach leaves

1 avocado, stone removed, peeled and sliced

1 chilli, finely sliced (leave the seeds in if you like the heat)

2 tablespoons extra virgin olive oil

½ lemon, juice only

salt and black pepper

For the lemony mayonnaise

1 heaped tablespoon mayonnaise (homemade (page 234) or shop-bought) with some lemon juice stirred in

Heat the butter in a frying pan on a medium heat and when it starts to become nutty and turn brown, add the sardines, skin side down.

Cook for around 4 minutes, until the skin is crisp and the flesh starts to become opaque, then remove from the pan and allow to rest for a minute or two (it will continue to cook a bit more as it rests).

If using tinned sardines there is no need to cook them.

Divide the leaves and avocado between two plates and top with the sardines. Scatter over the chilli and drizzle over the oil and lemon juice.

Season to taste and serve immediately, with the lemony mayonnaise on the side.

Sardine and roast pepper salad

Serves 2

Takes 10 minutes

The salty umami of the sardines on a bed of fresh green salad leaves, sweet roasted peppers and filling white beans makes a vibrant, delicious salad. More assembly job than cooking, its simple preparation belies its fresh and tasty goodness.

135g tin of sardines in extra virgin olive oil, oil reserved

400g tin of white beans, drained and rinsed

1 romaine lettuce, shredded

50g rocket leaves

4 roasted peppers from a jar (or roast your own), torn

10 cherry tomatoes, halved

salt and black pepper

For the dressing

2 tablespoons extra virgin olive oil, plus the oil from the tin of sardines

1 lemon, juice only

1 clove of garlic, finely grated

¼ teaspoon smoked paprika

2 teaspoons chopped parsley

To serve

lemon wedges

Drain the sardines, reserving the oil. Snip them into chunks with kitchen scissors and keep to one side.

Tip the white beans into a sieve or colander over the sink, then wash the beans under the cold tap for about 30 seconds, gently shaking, until the water draining through runs clear. Turn off the tap and allow to drain thoroughly to remove excess water.

Put the salad leaves into a mixing bowl or lunchbox, add the peppers, white beans and tomatoes, and toss everything together.

Mix the dressing by whisking everything together in a small bowl or shaking everything together in a clean jam jar. If eating away from home, carry the dressing in a watertight container and dress just before eating. If eating at home, pour the dressing over the salad and toss to coat.

Top the salad with the sardines and season to taste. Serve with fresh lemon wedges to squeeze over the sardines and some more salad leaves if you like.

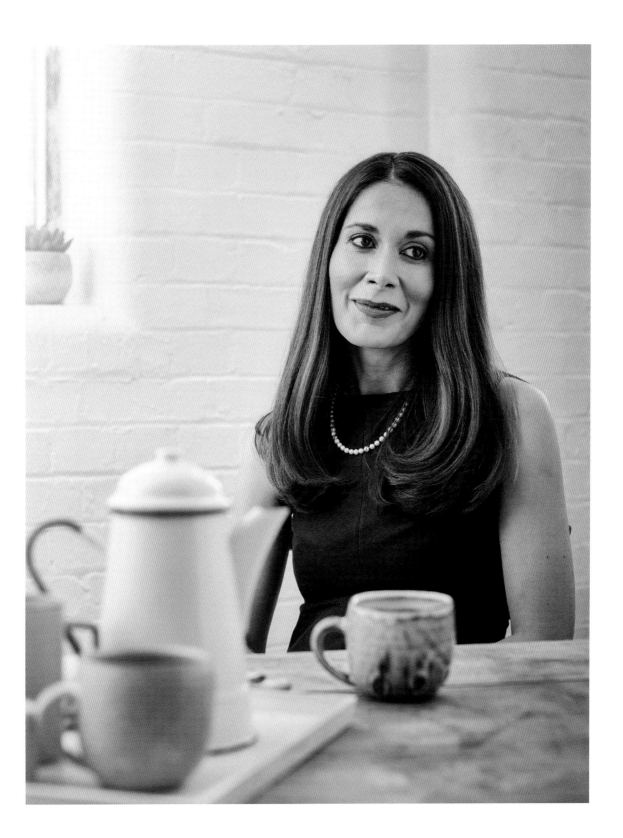

Error

Mackerel with beetroot and fennel salad

Serves 2

Takes 20 minutes

The crisp goodness of the mackerel, full of healthy fish oils, is perfect served resting on a bed of sweet beetroot, mixed with fresh herbs suffused with the liquorice flavour of fennel.

For the mackerel

1 tablespoon olive oil

4 uncooked mackerel fillets (these often come in packs of 2)

salt and black pepper

For the salad

1 large beetroot, peeled and grated

1 small fennel, very thinly sliced

40g watercress

1 tablespoon finely chopped dill

For the dressing

2 tablespoons extra virgin olive oil

1 tablespoon white wine vinegar

1 teaspoon wholegrain mustard

salt and black pepper

Rub the olive oil over the mackerel fillets and season with salt and pepper.

Heat a non-stick frying pan over a high heat and add the fillets skin side down. Cook for 2–3 minutes, until the flesh starts to become opaque. You will need to gently press the fillets down with a spatula, as the heat will make them arch away from the pan.

Flip the fish and cook for 1 more minute until fully cooked through, then remove from the pan and allow the fish to rest.

Put the beetroot, fennel, watercress and dill into a large mixing bowl.

In a bowl or a clean jam jar, make the dressing by mixing together the olive oil, vinegar, mustard and seasoning.

Add the dressing to the salad and toss to combine. Divide between two serving plates and top with the mackerel fillets.

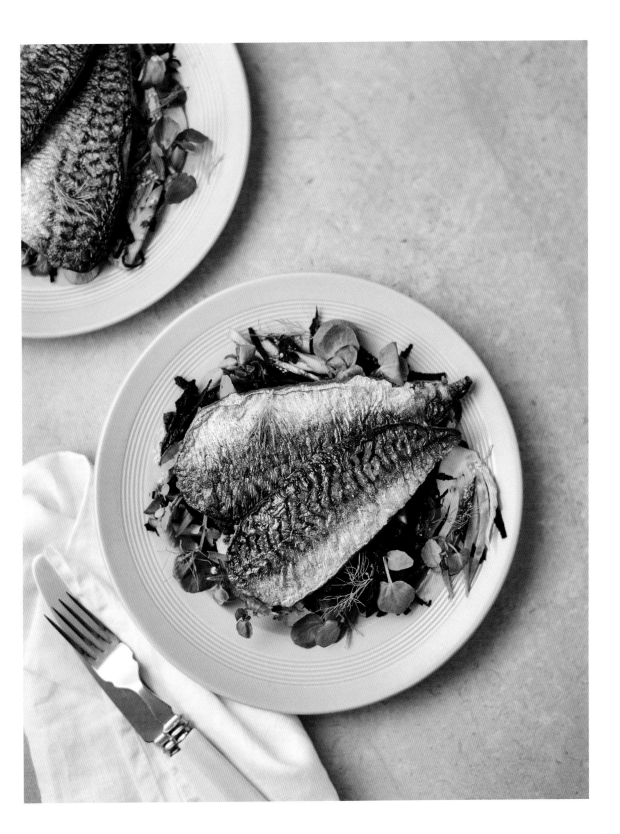

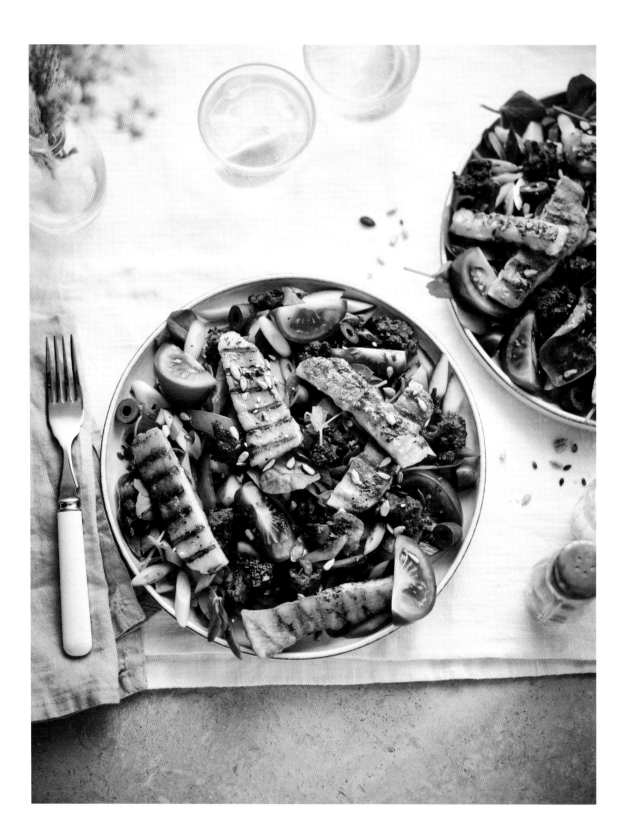

Chorizo and halloumi salad

Serves 2

Takes 20 minutes

I sometimes wonder if the hot, fatty, salty goodness of halloumi is unrivalled, and then I think of adding chorizo too! What's even more magic about this dish is that as the smoky fat of the chorizo releases, it coats the halloumi. The chorizo fat also forms the basis of the hot salad dressing, perfectly cut through by the acid zing of the fresh lemon.

100g cooking chorizo, peeled and cut into chunks

250g block of halloumi, cut into 6–8 slices depending on how thick you like it

For the salad

60g mixed salad leaves

1 green pepper (or colour of your choice), deseeded and cut into chunks

¼ cucumber, cut into chunks

2 ripe tomatoes, cut into wedges

6 spring onions, thinly sliced on the diagonal (optional)

12 black olives, pitted

For the dressing

1 lemon, juice to taste

1 teaspoon dried oregano

salt and black pepper

To serve

1 tablespoon mixed seeds

Heat a frying pan on a medium high heat and add the chopped chorizo. Once it has started to render some fat, tip the pan to coat the base in the oil. Add the slices of halloumi (you might need to do this in two batches) and cook them in the chorizo fat for 2–3 minutes each side, until golden.

When the halloumi and the chorizo caramelize and go sticky, remove from the pan and set to one side. Turn the heat off and reserve the oil in the pan for the dressing.

Put the salad leaves, pepper, cucumber, tomato, spring onions and olives into a large mixing bowl and toss to combine.

Add some lemon juice to the chorizo oil in the pan, along with the oregano and some seasoning. You may need to add a splash of extra virgin olive oil, depending on how much oil you have left from the chorizo. Whisk together in the pan and taste – you might need more lemon juice – then drizzle the dressing over your salad and toss.

Add the chorizo and halloumi, toss again, and top with a sprinkling of mixed seeds. Serve immediately, while the halloumi and chorizo are still hot.

Falafel salad

 Vegan

Serves 2

Takes 40 minutes

Whether it's the freshness of the herbs or the melting goodness of the hot chickpeas, there is something pleasingly satisfying about a falafel. Delicious served on a crunchy salad, these falafels are also ideal for dipping into hummus or tzatziki.

For the falafels

2 tablespoons olive oil

400g tin of chickpeas, drained and rinsed

4 spring onions, roughly chopped

1 tablespoon chopped coriander

1 tablespoon chopped parsley

1 clove of garlic, peeled

½ teaspoon ground coriander

½ teaspoon ground cumin

½ teaspoon baking powder

1 tablespoon sesame seeds

For the salad

½ romaine lettuce, shredded

¼ red cabbage, shredded

2 tomatoes, cut into chunks

¼ cucumber, cut into chunks

4 pickled chillies, sliced (check there's no added sugar)

For the dressing

1 tablespoon pow-pow! chilli sauce (page 237) (use more if you like) or if you don't have the pow-pow! to hand use Tabasco Red Pepper Hot Sauce instead, ½ teaspoon to start, and add more to taste

Preheat the oven to 200°C/180°C fan/gas 6. Line a baking tin with non-stick baking paper and use a little of the olive oil to grease the paper.

Put half the chickpeas into a mini chopper or a food processor with the spring onions, herbs, garlic, coriander, cumin and baking powder, and blitz to a rough paste. Add the rest of the chickpeas and pulse just until they are broken into the mix. Divide the mix into 8 even amounts and use your hands to shape them into flat patties.

Lay the falafels on the prepared baking tray, sprinkle the sesame seeds over the top and gently press the seeds down into the falafels. Drizzle over the remaining olive oil and bake in the oven for 20 minutes. Remove the tin from the oven, turn the falafels over, and return to the oven for another 10 minutes until they are crisp on the outside.

Put all the ingredients for the salad into a mixing bowl and toss to combine.

Whisk together the ingredients for the dressing (if it's a little thick, add a splash of water), pour over the salad and toss well. If eating away from home, carry the dressing in a watertight container and dress before eating. Divide the salad between two plates or add a portion to a lunchbox and top each one with 4 falafels.

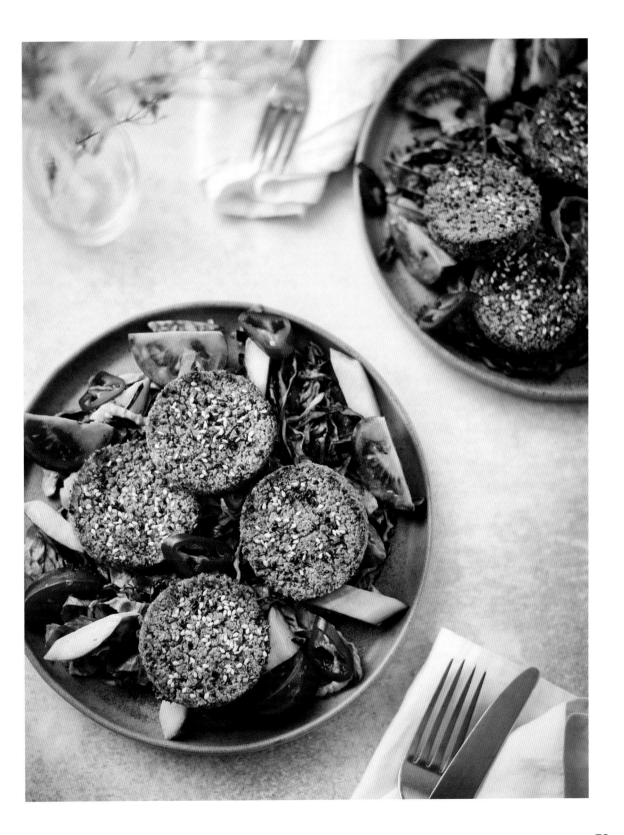

Chilled avocado soup

Serves 2

Takes 15 minutes, plus chilling time (this can be reduced if everything is in the fridge to start with)

2 avocados, halved and flesh scooped out

1 cucumber, peeled, seeds removed, cut into chunks

1 lemon, juice only

150ml vegetable stock (either homemade (page 259) or shop-bought fresh stock is also a good option if you can't find a stock cube with straightforward-sounding ingredients)

150ml natural full-fat yoghurt

salt and black pepper

To serve

1 red chilli, deseeded and finely chopped

1 teaspoon chopped chives or coriander

black pepper

super seeded crackers, crumbled (page 230) (optional)

There is something unexpected and particularly refreshing about a cold soup. Ideal for a hot summer's day, with a perfect blend of creamy avocado richness cut through by the simple freshness of the cucumber and the acid zing of the lemon juice, this chilled soup is a bowl of cooling green goodness.

Put the avocado, cucumber, lemon juice, vegetable stock and yoghurt into a food processor with some salt and pepper, and blitz for a few minutes until smooth. You can also blitz in a bowl using a stick blender if preferred. If you want the soup thinner, add a splash more stock.

Pour through a sieve into a bowl below, and chill in the fridge for at least an hour.

Divide between two bowls and top with chillies, chives or coriander and some more black pepper. You could also crumble in a few super seeded crackers for some extra crouton crunch.

Roast red pepper and tomato soup

 Vegan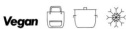

Serves 4

Takes 1 hour

Hands-on: 10 minutes
Hands-off: 50 minutes

Perfect to eat at home or to carry in a warming flask on the go — you can batch cook for extra convenience and freeze for future use so it's readily available anytime you feel like a meal of sweet and smoky goodness.

4 red peppers, deseeded and cut into chunks

6 ripe tomatoes, cut into chunks

1 red onion, cut into chunks

2 tablespoons olive oil

1 tablespoon dried oregano

2 teaspoons smoked paprika

5 cloves of garlic, peeled and crushed

1 litre vegetable stock (either homemade (page 259) or or shop-bought fresh stock is also a good option if you can't find a stock cube with straightforward-sounding ingredients)

200ml double cream (optional)

salt and black pepper

To serve

extra virgin olive oil

basil leaves

mixed seeds, such as sunflower or pumpkin

Preheat the oven to 200°C/180°C fan/gas 6.

Line a large roasting tin with baking paper and add the peppers, tomatoes and onion. Drizzle over the olive oil and add the oregano, paprika and some seasoning. Toss to coat the vegetables, then roast for 20 minutes. Briefly remove from the oven, turn everything, add the garlic and stir to combine, then return to the oven and roast for another 20 minutes.

Remove the roasted vegetables from the oven, transfer to a saucepan and add the stock. Bring to a simmer, then remove from the heat and use a stick blender or transfer to the bowl of a food processor and blitz until smooth.

Check the seasoning and consistency. Add more salt and pepper if you like. If you like it thicker, simply return the soup to the hob and simmer for 10–15 minutes — or if you prefer it looser, add a splash of water.

Add the cream and stir through. Leave out this step for a vegan option.

To serve, add a splash of extra virgin olive oil and garnish with a few fresh basil leaves and a sprinkle of mixed seeds.

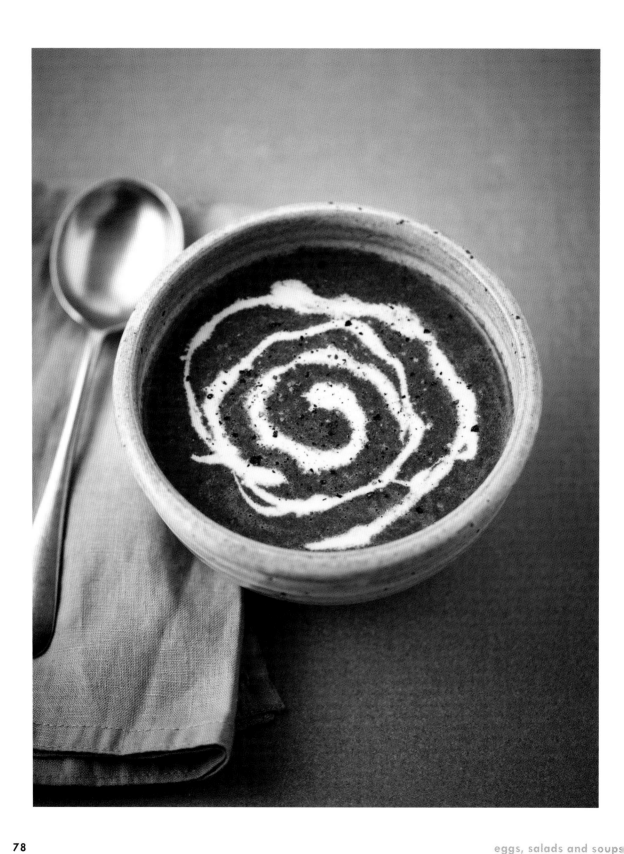

Cream of spinach soup

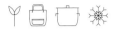

Serves 2

Takes 30 minutes

Hands-on: 10 minutes
Hands-off: 20 minutes

2 tablespoons olive oil

1 onion, peeled and chopped

2 sticks of celery, chopped

1 carrot, peeled and
  chopped

3 cloves of garlic, peeled
  and finely grated

½ teaspoon ground or
  freshly grated nutmeg

250g spinach leaves

200ml vegetable stock
  (homemade (page 259) or
  shop-bought fresh stock is
  also a good option if you
  can't find a stock cube with
  straightforward-sounding
  ingredients)

300ml whole milk

50–100ml double cream

salt and black pepper

There's a green glory about this velvety smooth, creamy soup, infused with the mineral goodness of the spinach. Delicious served piping hot from the pot, either in a bowl or in a large mug to wrap your hands around on a cold day.

Heat the oil in a large saucepan and add the onion, celery and carrot. Cook on a medium heat for around 10 minutes, until softened, and without catching too much colour. Add the garlic and stir through.

Add the nutmeg and spinach and stir until the spinach just starts to wilt. Then add the stock and milk and cook for 10 minutes, until the spinach has wilted right down. Turn off the heat and use a stick blender to blend until smooth, or alternatively pour into the bowl of a food processor and blitz. If you want a very smooth soup, place a sieve on top of a large bowl and pour the soup through the sieve into the bowl below.

Add as much of the cream as you need to get the consistency you like, reserving some for serving.

Season to taste, add a final swirl of cream on top and serve while hot.

Roast chickpea and cauliflower soup

Serves 4

Takes 55 minutes

Hands-on: 15 minutes
Hands-off: 40 minutes

2 x 400g tins of chickpeas, drained and rinsed

1 small cauliflower, cut into florets

1 onion, peeled and sliced

1 carrot, peeled and cut into chunks

4 cloves of garlic, peeled and crushed

3 tablespoons olive oil

1 teaspoon ground cumin

1 teaspoon ground coriander

1 teaspoon ground turmeric

½ teaspoon chilli powder

1 litre vegetable stock (use homemade (page 259) or shop-bought, fresh stock is also a good option if you can't find a stock cube with straightforward-sounding ingredients)

2 tablespoons crème fraîche

2 tablespoons chopped coriander

salt and black pepper

super seeded crackers (page 230)

The nuttiness of the roasted chickpeas sings in this warming, golden, velvety rich cauliflower soup. Ideal to eat at home or carried on the go in a flask, and delicious served with super seeded crackers (page 230) for that satisfying extra crunch.

Preheat the oven to 180°C/160°C fan/gas 4 and line two roasting tins with baking paper.

Tip the chickpeas out of the tin into a sieve or colander set over the sink, then rinse under the cold tap until the water draining out runs clear, which usually takes about 30 seconds.

Divide the chickpeas, cauliflower, onion, carrot and garlic between the two roasting tins. In a small bowel or jug, mix the olive oil and spices, then pour over the chickpeas and vegetables and toss to coat.

Roast in the oven for around 30 minutes, until golden brown, stirring once halfway through. Then remove from the oven and reserving around half of the chickpea mixture from one of the roasting tins, tip the rest into a large saucepan. Add the vegetable stock and bring to a simmer. Cook for 10 minutes.

Turn off the heat, then use a stick blender to blitz the soup until smooth, or alternatively transfer to a food processor and blitz. Season to taste and add a little water if you prefer your soup a bit looser.

Add the crème fraîche and stir through. Stir in the chopped coriander. Add some of the reserved crispy roasted chickpeas and a twist of black pepper. Check the seasoning and serve while hot. Enjoy with a side of super seeded crackers (page 230) for some pleasing extra dunking crunch.

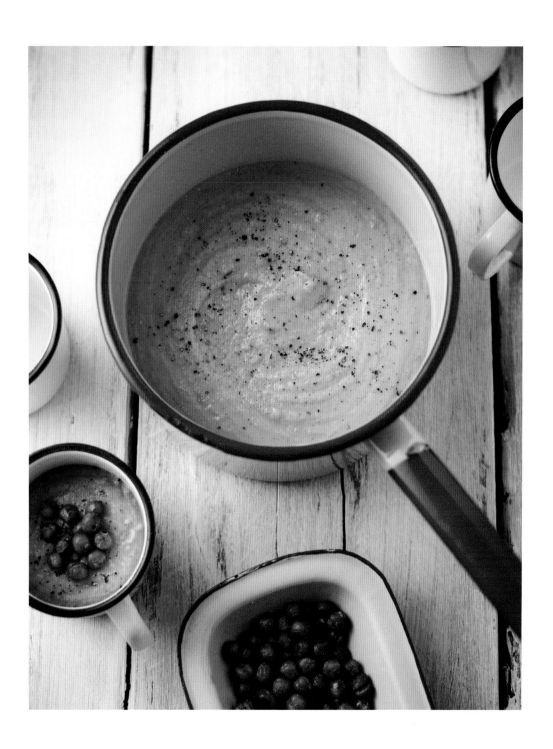

meat, fish and big veg

These delicious, big-ticket meals are full of flavour, nourishment and good eating. As with all the recipes, they are low sugar (to control insulin levels), contain essential healthy fats and generate a strong gut-to-brain fullness signal.

On the whole, these dishes take slightly longer to prepare, although many have a fair amount of 'hands-off' time too, which means that the dish takes care of itself – simmering, roasting or baking – while you are free to do something else. For even more time efficiency, many can be batch cooked and also freeze well too, so that cooking in the here and now sets you up beautifully for future meals.

Do also keep in mind that rather than eating for one, you are in fact eating for one hundred trillion – your gut bacteria. These dishes contain plenty of phytonutrients as well as prebiotics like fibre, for your gut bacteria to turn into substances that keep you feeling full.

The serving sizes are usually for more than one person, because if you live with or eat with other people, they will undoubtedly enjoy eating this food too. As with all the serving sizes in the book, do adjust the quantities to make more or less depending on your own situation.

That these recipes can be happily shared with others, whether or not they are looking to lose weight, emphasizes that, rather than being 'diet' food, these dishes are simply a healthy and delicious way to eat. My patients tell me time and again, that a great joy of the Programme is eating in the same way as the other people at your table, while at the same time moving ever forward towards your weight-loss and wellbeing goals.

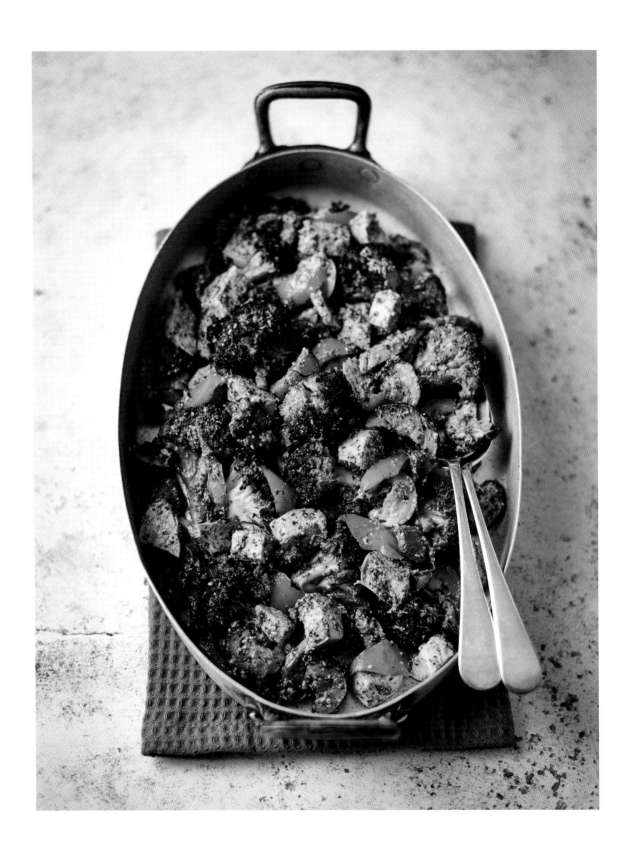

Pesto chicken and veg one-pan roast

Serves 2

Takes 45 minutes

Hands-on: 5 minutes
Hands-off: 40 minutes

160g roast chicken, roughly chopped (a good use for leftovers)

1 large pepper (colour of your choice), deseeded and cut into chunks

2 courgettes, cut into chunks

6 big broccoli florets

12 cherry tomatoes

1 tablespoon olive oil

1 teaspoon dried oregano

salt and black pepper

For the pesto

50g pine nuts, toasted

25g fresh basil

75ml olive oil

1 small clove of garlic, crushed

2 tablespoons grated Parmesan

black pepper

To serve

a handful of salad leaves

This zingy, fresh pesto will lift any veg you want to use in this one-pan roast – a great way of using up leftovers – just throw it in and let the pesto work its magic! This super pesto will also be a versatile addition to your Full Diet repertoire – delicious as an accompaniment to meat and fish, a vegetable topping and a salad dressing – its green goodness goes a long way.

Preheat the oven to 170°C/150°C fan/gas 3 and line a roasting tin with baking paper.

Put the chicken into a mixing bowl and keep to one side.

Place all the vegetables in the roasting tin, drizzle over the olive oil and add the oregano and some seasoning. Toss the veg to coat and place in the hot oven for 40 minutes, turning the vegetables halfway through.

While the vegetables are roasting, you can make the pesto. First, toast the pine nuts by placing them in a frying pan or skillet over a medium heat for 2–3 minutes, shaking the pan frequently until the pine nuts just start to brown. Make sure to keep a close eye on them as they can burn easily.

Remove from the heat, then put the pine nuts, basil, olive oil and garlic into a mini chopper or food processor and blitz until quite smooth. Add the Parmesan and some black pepper and pulse to just combine. Keep to one side.

When the vegetables are done (you want them to be soft and golden), transfer them to the bowl containing the chicken. Add as much of the pesto as you like and toss to coat everything. Divide between two serving plates or lunchboxes. When ready to eat, you can add a handful of salad leaves too.

If you have leftover pesto it will keep in the fridge in an airtight container for a week; just cover it with a thin layer of olive oil.

Golden buttermilk chicken popcorn

Serves 2

Takes 40–50 minutes,
plus marinating time

Hands-on: 10–15 minutes
Hands-off: 30–35 minutes

400g chicken thighs, skinless
and boneless, each thigh cut
into 4 pieces

300ml buttermilk

1 teaspoon salt

250g mixed seeds (mix of
any of sunflower, pumpkin,
sesame, poppy or linseeds)

2 tablespoons dried mixed
herbs

olive oil, for drizzling

To serve (optional)

mayonnaise (homemade
(page 234) or shop-
bought), for dipping

Ultra-processed food gives nugget-style chicken a bad name.
Done The Full Diet way, they are nutritious and delicious, and the
crunchy seed coating is a great meal for your gut bacteria too.

Put the chopped chicken thighs into a large mixing bowl and add
the buttermilk and the salt. Mix really well to coat the chicken.
Cover and leave to marinate in the fridge overnight.

Preheat the oven to 190°C/170°C fan/gas 5 and line two baking
sheets with greaseproof paper.

While the oven is warming up, blitz the mixed seeds in a mini chopper
or food processor to roughly break them down to a coarse bread-
crumb-like consistency. Place the blitzed seeds and mixed herbs in a
shallow dish and combine well.

Take the chicken piece by piece and shake off most of the buttermilk.
Roll in the ground seed-herb mix until well coated, then place the
chicken on one of the lined baking sheets. Leave space around each
piece to avoid it getting sweaty rather than baking. Wash your
hands thoroughly after handling raw chicken.

Once all the chicken is coated and placed on the baking sheet,
drizzle a little olive oil over each piece.

Place the trays in the oven and after 20 minutes carefully turn the
chicken — the crumb is more delicate than on a regular nugget.

Return to the oven for another 15–20 minutes, until the nuggets are
crisp and brown. Season to taste.

Serve with a rocket salad or, steamed green beans, carrot and
poppy seed crunch (page 223), or any veg side of your choice.

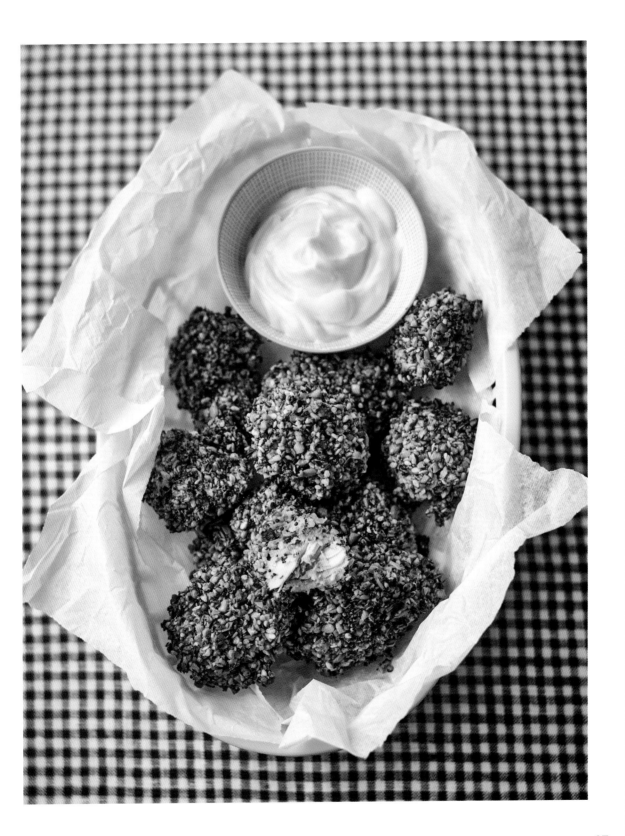

Butter chicken

Takes 1 hour
25 minutes, plus
marinating time

Hands-on:
25 minutes
Hands-off:
1 hour

This modern Indian classic combines a depth of spice flavour with the creamy goodness of the sauce to make this melt-in-the-mouth butter chicken a perennial favourite.

For the marinade

3 tablespoons full-fat
natural yoghurt

4 cloves of garlic,
peeled and finely
grated

3cm piece of ginger,
peeled and grated

2 teaspoons garam
masala

1 teaspoon ground
turmeric

1 teaspoon chilli
powder

1 lemon, juice only

For the curry

1kg chicken thighs,
skinless and
boneless, each thigh
cut into 6 chunks

40g butter or ghee

2 tablespoons olive
oil

1 onion, halved
and sliced

3 cloves of garlic,
peeled and finely
grated

1 red chilli, finely
chopped

1 teaspoon garam
masala

½ teaspoon ground
cardamom

8 curry leaves, fresh
or dried (optional)

3 tablespoons tomato
purée

100ml double cream

1 lemon, juice to taste

salt and black
pepper

Place all the ingredients for the marinade into a mixing bowl and whisk together. Add the chicken thighs and coat thoroughly in the marinade. Cover the bowl and refrigerate for a minimum of 4 hours but ideally overnight.

When you are ready to cook the chicken, heat the butter or ghee and olive oil in a large saucepan or casserole pot and when hot, add the onions, garlic and chilli. Cook for 5–10 minutes on a medium heat, until soft and starting to go golden.

Add the garam masala, cardamom, curry leaves and tomato purée and cook for a couple more minutes. Keep a close eye, as the spices can burn easily. Once the spices are lightly toasted, add the chicken and the marinade.

Cook for 10 minutes, then add the double cream and half the lemon juice, reserving the rest for serving. Turn the heat down low, cover the pan with a lid, and cook for another hour. Add a splash of water if it gets too thick, and stir every now and again to stop anything catching on the bottom of the pan. Once cooked, add seasoning to taste and a splash more lemon juice if you like.

Serve on a bed of deliciously nutty cauliflower rice (page 216).

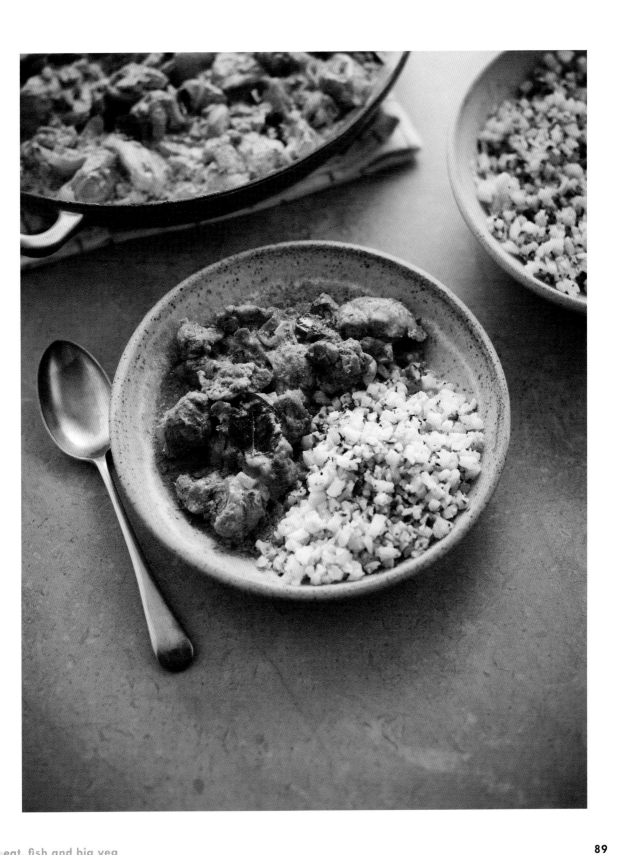

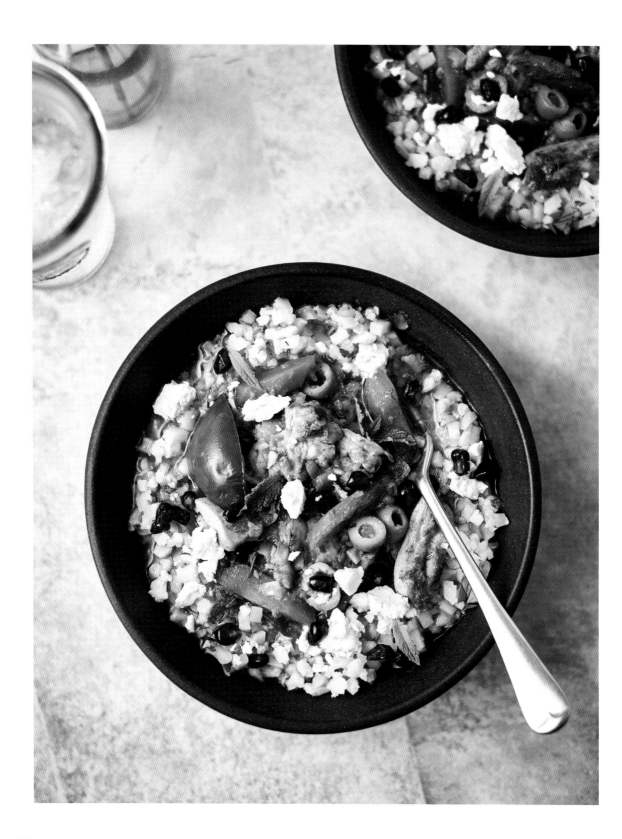

Chicken tagine

Serves 2

Takes 1 hour 20 minutes

Hands-on: 20 minutes
Hands-off: 1 hour

This fragrant tagine has a depth of rich flavour that infuses as the chicken slowly cooks. Serve this richly spiced Moroccan classic on a bed of cauliflower rice and adorn it with sweet pomegranate seeds, crumbled feta and fresh mint for extra bejewelled goodness.

2 tablespoons olive oil

1 onion, diced

2 carrots, peeled and cut into chunks

4 chicken thighs, skinless and boneless, each thigh cut into 6 pieces

3 cloves of garlic, peeled and finely grated

2cm piece of fresh ginger, peeled and grated

1 teaspoon ground coriander

1 teaspoon ground cumin

1 teaspoon fennel seeds

1 teaspoon ground black pepper

2 tomatoes, each cut into quarters

300ml chicken stock (homemade (pages 257–8) or shop-bought fresh chicken stock is also a good option if you can't find a stock cube with straightforward-sounding ingredients)

30g pitted green olives, halved

1 tablespoon chopped parsley

salt

To serve

pomegranate seeds

40g feta, crumbled

harissa

mint leaves

lemon wedges

Preheat the oven to 190°C/170°C fan/gas 5.

Heat the oil in a casserole pot and add the onion and carrot. Cook for 5 minutes on a medium high heat, until just starting to soften.

Add the chicken, garlic and ginger. Cook for another 5 minutes until the chicken is browned on all sides.

Add the spices, tomatoes and stock. Bring to a simmer, then cover the pot with a lid and cook in the oven for 45 minutes. Stir once, halfway through the cooking time.

Remove from the oven and take off the lid. Add the olives, then return the uncovered pot to the oven for another 15 minutes.

Remove from the oven and add a little salt, but taste as you season, as if you are using shop-bought stock this can be quite salty. Garnish with the parsley, then ladle the tagine on to a bed of cauliflower rice (page 216). Serve with pomegranate seeds, crumbled feta, harissa, mint leaves and lemon wedges for that final wow of colour and taste.

Tofu or chicken schnitzel with spring greens in a fresh tomato sauce

(if vegetarian Parmesan used)

Serves 2

Takes 20 minutes (plus pressing time if using tofu)

Pan-fried tofu or chicken coated in a tasty Parmesan-almond crumb makes a delicious take on this Austro-German classic. Serve with spring greens cooked in a fresh tomato sauce and cover with Parmesan for extra umami yum.

300g piece of firm tofu, cut into two 'steaks' (Dragonfly brand is excellent for this)

OR 2 skinless, boneless chicken breasts, flattened with a rolling pin to 1cm thick

2 tablespoons almond flour

1 egg, lightly beaten

1 tablespoon arrowroot powder

30g ground almonds

20g Parmesan, grated

1 teaspoon dried oregano

1 teaspoon sweet smoked paprika

olive oil

salt and black pepper

For the tomato sauce

680g jar of passata

2 cloves of garlic, peeled and finely grated

1 tablespoon chopped basil

200g spring greens, shredded

To serve

2 tablespoons grated Parmesan

If using tofu, start by pressing out the excess water. To do this, lay out some kitchen paper and place the two tofu steaks on it. Top with more kitchen paper, then place a heavy casserole pot (or other heavy object) on top. Press the tofu for at least 30 minutes, changing the paper frequently when it becomes wet.

Once the tofu is ready, set up three bowls: one with the almond flour, one with the beaten egg (or oat milk if using), and one with the arrowroot powder, ground almonds, Parmesan, oregano, paprika, salt and pepper, mixed together.

Dip the tofu into the almond flour, then into the beaten egg, and then into the ground almond mix. Repeat with the other slice.

Heat some olive oil in a frying pan and once hot, add the tofu. Cook for approximately 4–5 minutes each side until golden and crisp.

If using chicken, follow the same coating process described for the tofu. Wash your hands thoroughly after handling raw meat. Fry as above, cooking on a medium high heat. It should be done within 12–15 minutes.

While the tofu/chicken is cooking, put the passata, grated garlic and basil into a pan and cook for 5 minutes on a medium high heat to thicken slightly. Add the shredded spring greens and cook in the sauce for 5–6 minutes, until al dente.

Divide the greens between two serving plates, top each with a schnitzel and cover liberally with Parmesan. Eat immediately.

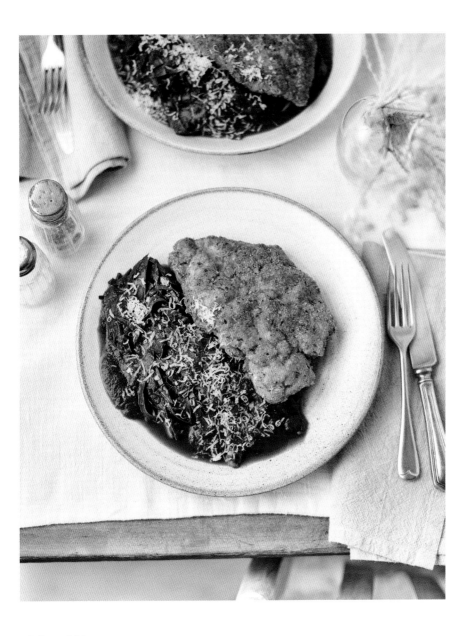

Aromatic lamb koftas with sumac salad

Serves 2

Takes 25 minutes

These fragrant koftas are bursting with flavour, with the warmth of the spices and the bite of the garlic lifting the sweet fattiness of the lamb. The fresh salad is the natural counterbalance to the richness of the meat. Perfect as a meal any time of year, these koftas are also brilliant on the barbecue – just increase the quantities depending on how many people are coming!

For the koftas

400g lamb mince

1 bunch of spring onions, finely chopped

2 tablespoons chopped fresh coriander

1 large clove of garlic, finely grated

½ teaspoon ground coriander

½ teaspoon ground cumin

½ teaspoon ground cinnamon

black pepper

For the salad

1 romaine lettuce or other lettuce of choice, chopped

12 cherry tomatoes or 2 tomatoes, quartered, then each quarter cut in half again

1 small red onion, thinly sliced (optional)

¼ cucumber, thinly sliced

1 tablespoon roughly chopped mint leaves

For the dressing

2 tablespoons full-fat Greek yoghurt

2 tablespoons extra virgin olive oil

½ lemon, juice only

1 tablespoon sumac

salt and black pepper

To serve

sumac

parsley leaves

Place all the ingredients for the koftas in a large mixing bowl and use your hands to really knead and work the mix together. This will take a few minutes. Alternatively, mix in an electric mixer for about 5 minutes, which will get them really well combined.

Divide the mix evenly into 6, then taking 6 skewers work the mix on to each skewer, shaping it into a rough sausage. Squeeze it tightly to mould it to the skewer to prevent meat falling off. Wash your hands thoroughly after handling raw meat.

Heat a large frying pan or griddle and place the skewers in the pan. Cook for around 2–3 minutes each side (around 8–12 minutes in total) until well coloured and cooked through. You can check this by making a small incision in one.

While the koftas are cooking, put the lettuce, tomatoes, onion (if using), cucumber and mint leaves into a salad bowl. To make the dressing, put the yoghurt, extra virgin olive oil, lemon juice and sumac into a jug and whisk to combine (or use a clean jam jar and shake it all together).

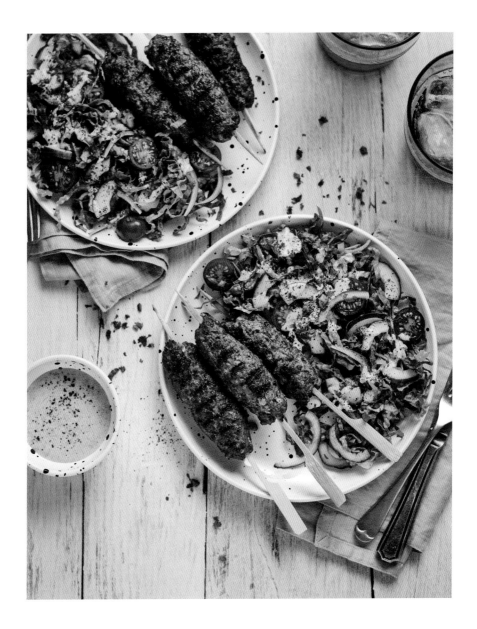

Season to taste, and add more lemon if you like it sharper or a little more yoghurt for a creamier dressing. Add half the dressing to the salad leaves and toss to coat.

Divide the salad between two plates and top each one with 3 koftas. Drizzle over a little more dressing, and add an extra sprinkle of sumac and some parsley leaves. Serve with extra dressing on the side for dipping.

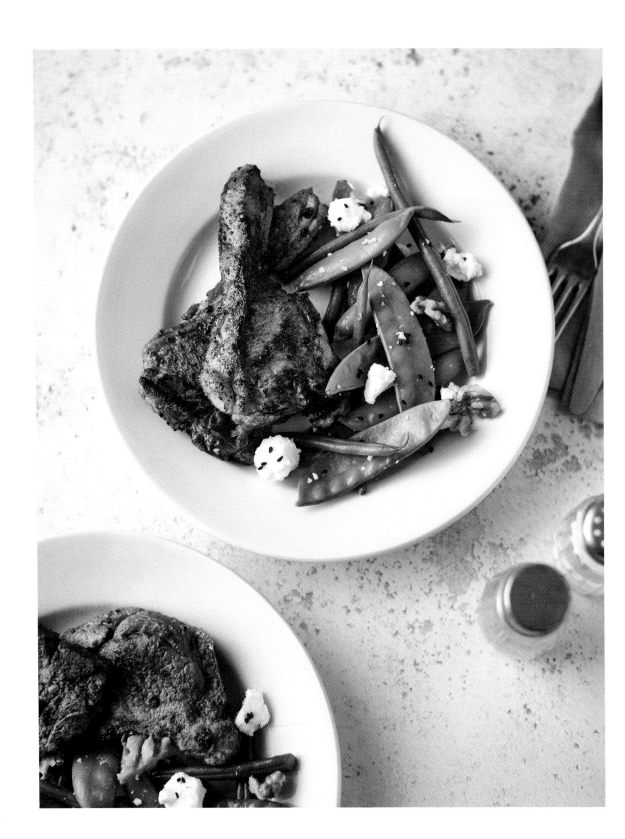

Herb and garlic lamb chops

Serves 2

Takes 25 minutes,
plus marinating time

6 lamb chops

2 tablespoons olive oil

½ lemon, juice only

3 tablespoons roughly chopped
fresh parsley

2 tablespoons thyme leaves

2 cloves of garlic, peeled and
roughly sliced

black pepper

To serve

lemon wedges

Delicious, sweet lamb, singing in a marinade of fresh herbs and garlic, cut through with the acid clarity of lemon juice, this recipe has been a Programme favourite group after group. Delicious with some hummus on the side or some feta cheese crumbled on top, or just left as is. This also works really well for a summer barbecue.

Place the chops in a tub with a lid that can hold them all snugly — a Tupperware-type container works very well.

Pour the olive oil and lemon juice into a mini chopper or the small bowl of a food processor and add the parsley, thyme, garlic and some black pepper. Blitz to a coarse paste and tip over the lamb chops.

Put the lid on the container and shake vigorously to coat the chops in the herb mixture, then chill in the fridge for a minimum of 6 hours.

Remove the chops from the fridge about an hour before cooking, to bring them up to room temperature.

Heat a frying pan or griddle pan and place the chops fat edges down in the pan, all tightly packed together, over a low heat. You want to render the fat slowly over about 10 minutes. Check occasionally that they're not burning, but try to leave them as much as possible.

Once the fat is deliciously golden and crisp, lay the chops down on one side. Cook for 2–3 minutes, then flip and cook the other side for 2–3 minutes (the cooking time will depend on how pink you like your chops).

Remove from the heat and allow to rest for a few minutes before serving. Serve with a wedge of lemon to squeeze over the chops at the table.

Delicious served with steamed green beans, broccoli mash (page 218) or super crunchy rainbow slaw (page 202). Also works well with a tablespoon of hummus on the side to dip into.

Moussaka

Serves 6

Takes 1 hour 15 minutes

Hands-on: 45 minutes
Hands-off: 30 minutes

If you liked the aubergine parmigiana in *The Full Diet*, you'll love this riff on a similar theme – fragrant lamb, layered with aubergine and crowned with a creamy rich béchamel. It's delicious eaten bubbling straight from the oven, brilliantly complemented by the fiery peppery freshness of the rocket.

1 tablespoon olive oil

1 onion, diced

2 carrots, peeled and diced

3 sticks of celery, diced

3 tablespoons tomato purée

4 cloves of garlic, peeled and finely grated

800g lamb mince

2 tablespoons dried oregano

2 teaspoons ground cinnamon

2 x 400g tins of chopped tomatoes

salt and black pepper

For the layers

2 large aubergines, peeled and cut into 5mm thick slices

3 tablespoons olive oil

1 large courgette, cut into 5mm thick slices on the diagonal (to make them longer)

For the béchamel

280g cream cheese

300ml double cream

2 eggs

½ teaspoon ground or freshly grated nutmeg

200g halloumi, grated

To serve

rocket leaves

1 lemon, juice only

olive oil

Heat the oil in a large saucepan and add the onion, carrots and celery. Cook gently on a medium heat for about 10 minutes, until the vegetables are soft and just starting to go golden brown.

Add the tomato purée and cook for 1 minute, stirring to coat the vegetables, then add the garlic and cook for a further minute.

Add the lamb mince and increase the heat. Break the mince up, and cook for 10 minutes until the meat is browned. Stir frequently to cook evenly.

Add the oregano, cinnamon and chopped tomatoes and season with salt and lots of black pepper. Mix well and leave to cook gently on a medium heat while you prepare everything else (around 15–20 minutes).

Heat a large frying pan on a high heat and add as many aubergine slices as will fit easily. Once you see them just starting to go brown, add a drizzle of the olive oil all over and turn the slices. Keep turning every now and again until they are a deep golden brown and soft all through. Carefully transfer the aubergines to a large plate or chopping board lined with kitchen paper to absorb any excess oil. Repeat with all the other aubergine slices and then with the courgette.

To make the béchamel, whisk the cream cheese, double cream, eggs, nutmeg, some seasoning and half the grated halloumi together in a large jug or mixing bowl, using a fork.

Preheat the oven to 200°C/180°C fan/gas 6.

To assemble, place a quarter of the lamb mince mix in the base of a roasting dish that's about 35cm x 20cm. Top with a layer of the aubergine, then another layer of the lamb, then the courgette, then more lamb, then the remaining aubergine. Top with the rest of the lamb and smooth right down.

Pour the béchamel all over the top and place the roasting dish in the oven for 15 minutes. Take the dish out and sprinkle over the rest of the grated halloumi, then cook for another 20–30 minutes, until bubbling and golden brown. The top should have set and risen.

Remove from the oven. Plate up generous handfuls of rocket leaves, drizzle over some lemon juice and olive oil and serve the moussaka alongside.

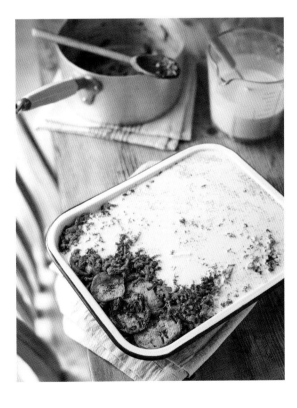
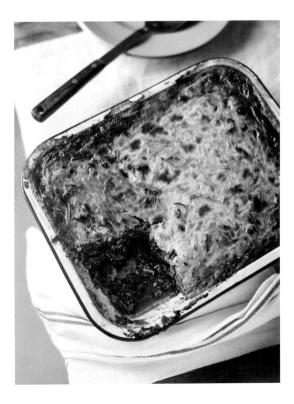

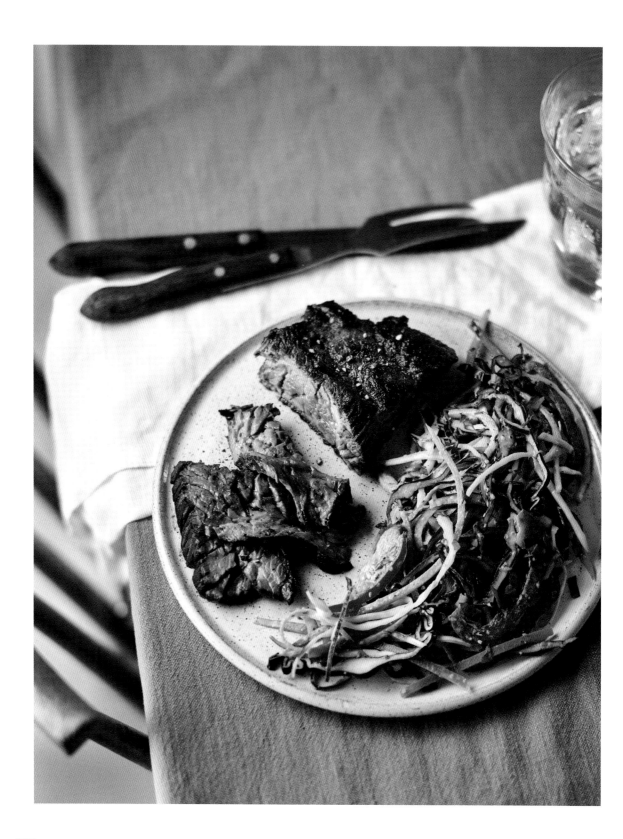

Steak and piri-piri slaw

Serves 2

Takes 30 minutes

Choose whichever cut of steak you like best or one that's on offer — all cuts work well with this tasty creamy slaw, which is also a delicious side to many of the recipes in this book and ideal for summer picnics and barbecues. Dial up the heat of the slaw as high as you like, or you might sometimes want to leave out the piri-piri for a more mellow slaw — as always, it's up to you.

2 steaks, cut of your choice (each approx. 200g)

For the piri-piri seasoning

2 tablespoons sweet smoked paprika

2 tablespoons garlic powder

1 tablespoon onion powder

1 tablespoon dried oregano

1–3 teaspoons cayenne pepper (depending on how hot you want it)

2 teaspoons ground coriander

1 teaspoon ground cardamom

1 teaspoon ground or freshly grated nutmeg

For the slaw

1 large carrot, peeled and julienned (cut into long thin batons)

¼ small white cabbage and ½ small red cabbage, both thinly sliced on a mandolin, with a knife or using the grater attachment of a food processor

¼ red onion, sliced very thinly into a crescent moon shape (optional)

1 tablespoon piri-piri seasoning (see above)

2 tablespoons mayonnaise (homemade (page 234) or shop-bought)

2 tablespoons roughly chopped fresh coriander

1 red pepper, deseeded and thinly sliced (optional)

juice of 1 lemon (to taste)

salt and black pepper

Remove the steaks from the fridge, take them out of their packaging, and pat dry with kitchen paper. Keep covered with the kitchen paper and leave them for an hour before cooking, to allow the steaks to come up to room temperature.

To make the piri-piri seasoning, simply shake everything together in a Tupperware-style container. This makes more than you need, but it will keep for 3–6 months.

For the slaw, put all the ingredients into a large mixing bowl and stir well to combine. Check for seasoning and add more lemon juice if needed. Leave to one side while you cook the steaks.

Heat a frying pan and when really hot, add the steaks. As a guide for a 200g steak, cook for 1½ minutes each side for rare, 2 minutes on each side for medium/rare, 2½ minutes on each side for medium and 3 to 3½ minutes on each side for well done. You can cut through the steak to check how it is cooked and can briefly return to the pan if you feel it needs extra cooking time although, it will also cook a bit more while it is resting.

Remove from the pan and allow to rest for a few minutes.

Slice the steaks, check the seasoning and serve with the piri-piri slaw on the side.

Satay beef with crunchy slaw

Serves 2

Takes 25 minutes

The spicy, salty creaminess of the satay sauce and crunchy slaw bring intense layers of flavour to the beef. The satay sauce is also delicious with chicken and the slaw works brilliantly as a side with any other dish of your choosing.

2 sirloin steaks (or your choice of cut, e.g. rump, bavette, rib-eye), cut into 2cm cubes (approx. 200g each)

For the satay sauce

4 teaspoons crunchy peanut butter (make sure its palm oil free and there's no added sugar)

2 tablespoons full-fat natural yoghurt (or Greek yoghurt)

100ml coconut cream (check for any dubious ingredients)

1 lime, juice only

½ teaspoon chilli flakes (more if you like)

For the crunchy slaw

1 large carrot, peeled and julienned (cut into long thin batons)

¼ small white cabbage and ¼ small red cabbage, both thinly sliced on a mandolin, with a knife or using the grater attachment of a food processor

50g sugar snap peas, thinly sliced

50g mangetout, cut into bite-size pieces

4 spring onions, very thinly sliced

½ lime, juice only

1 tablespoon mayonnaise (homemade (page 234) or shop-bought)

sea salt and black pepper

Take the steaks out of the fridge about an hour before cooking, pat dry with kitchen paper and keep covered until ready to use.

Cut the steaks into 2cm cubes and thread on to 4 short skewers and keep to one side until you're ready to cook.

Place all the ingredients for the satay sauce in a mixing bowl and whisk together. It will make a loose dressing. Keep to one side.

For the slaw, put all the veg into a mixing bowl and toss to combine. Add the lime juice (more if you like), the mayonnaise and season to taste. Keep to one side.

Heat a large frying pan, griddle pan or barbecue and when hot add the skewers, with a little space around each one. Cook for 2 minutes each side for medium; a little less if you like medium rare and a little more if you want it well done.

Plate up 2 skewers per person, spoon over some of the satay sauce and serve alongside the slaw. Serve the remaining satay sauce on the table, to add more during the meal if wanted.

If there is any leftover satay sauce you can keep it in the fridge for up to a week – it's delicious with grilled chicken.

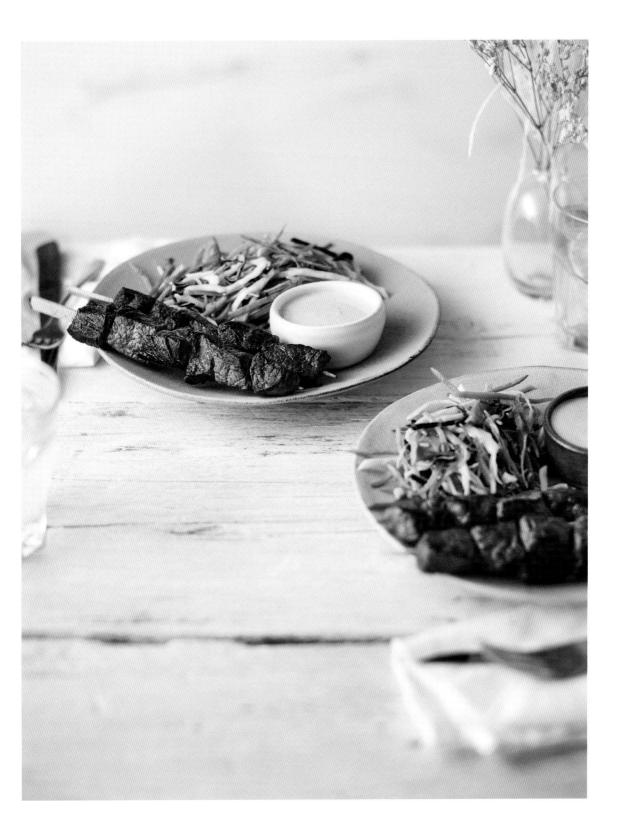

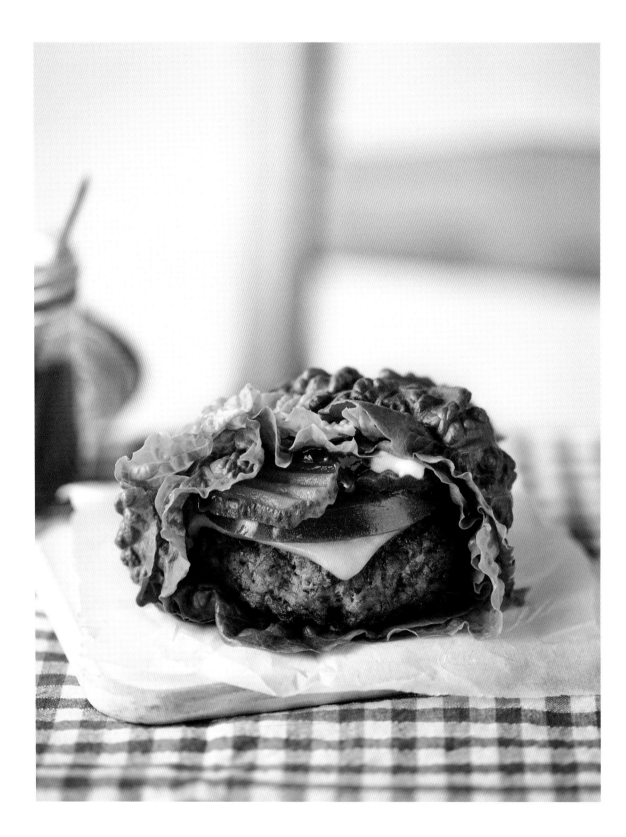

meat, fish and big ve

The 'good stuff' cheeseburgers

Seves 2

Takes 30 minutes

One of my patients once explained how, with The Full Diet way of eating, 'I only eat the good stuff!' This recipe is a perfect example of that philosophy because it's the burger that's the main event – not a bun. This recipe still includes the finger food experience of a traditional cheeseburger, but wrapped in a crispy, fresh lettuce leaf, which allows the star of the show – the burger – to shine through! Ideal cooked indoors as well as being brilliant for barbecues. Delicious served with super crunchy rainbow slaw (page 202).

For the burgers

400g beef mince (ideally around 15% fat)

2 tablespoons whole milk

1 teaspoon dried mixed herbs

½ teaspoon black pepper

To serve

4 slices of cheese of your choice (Cheddar, mozzarella, etc.)

8 lettuce leaves (iceberg, romaine, etc. all work well)

1 beef tomato, sliced

8 slices of dill pickle

fresh homemade ketchup (page 236)

mayonnaise (homemade (page 234) or shop-bought)

Put all the ingredients for the burgers into a mixing bowl and use your hands to really work the mix and combine everything well.

Shape the mix into 4 patties and chill until needed. Wash your hands thoroughly after handling raw meat.

When you are ready to eat the burgers, take them out of the fridge for about 15 minutes before cooking.

Heat a frying pan and when it's really hot add the burgers. Cook for around 4 minutes on each side, or to your liking.

With 2 minutes left to go, add the slices of cheese and cover the pan with a lid so the heat from the pan helps melt the cheese.

To assemble, take a lettuce leaf and place it on your plate. Top with one of the cheeseburgers, a slice of tomato, 2 slices of pickle and some ketchup or mayo, then add the lettuce topper. Serve each person 2 cheeseburgers.

These burgers are delicious served with celeriac chips (page 220).

Pork and pistachio meatballs with red cabbage and fennel braise

Serves 4

Takes 45 minutes, plus chilling time

Hands-on: 30 minutes
Hands-off: 15 minutes

Sweet green pistachios tucked into fragrantly spiced pork, resting on a bed of fennel-infused red cabbage – these warming meatballs are packed with flavourful goodness.

For the meatballs

500g pork mince (approx. 15% fat)

100g pistachios, shelled and finely chopped

2 cloves of garlic, peeled and finely grated

2 tablespoons finely chopped parsley

3 teaspoons onion powder

3 teaspoons sumac

black pepper

olive oil, for frying

For the vegetables

15g butter

1 tablespoon olive oil

1 red onion, peeled and thinly sliced

½ red cabbage, thinly sliced or shredded in a food processor

1 fennel, thinly sliced

300ml (approx.) vegetable stock, to cover (you can use homemade stock (page 259) or shop-bought fresh stock is also a good option if you can't find a stock cube with straightforward-sounding ingredients)

1 unwaxed lemon, zest and juice

salt and black pepper

To serve

soft fresh herbs, such as dill and/or parsley

200g full-fat Greek or natural yogurt with 1 tablespoon horseradish sauce (check there is no added sugar) or 2 tablespoons fresh herbs like parsley or dill stirred in

To make the meatballs, place all the ingredients apart from the olive oil in a mixing bowl and use your hands to combine them. Really work the mixture to break down the mince and get everything evenly distributed.

Divide into 12 even balls and shape into rounds. Place the meatballs on a plate and cover with clingfilm. Wash your hands thoroughly after handling raw meat. Chill the meatballs in the fridge for 30 minutes before cooking. When you want to cook them, remove them from the fridge 15 minutes before so that you aren't cooking them from fridge cold.

While the meatballs are chilling, heat the butter and olive oil in a sauté pan or frying pan on a medium heat. Add the red onion and cook for 10 minutes, until starting to soften. Then add the cabbage and fennel and cook for another 10 minutes.

Add the vegetable stock and lemon zest and bring to a simmer. Cook until the liquid has all but gone and the vegetables are tender but still have a bit of crunch, stirring occasionally so nothing catches. Finish with a squeeze of lemon juice and season to taste.

While the vegetables are simmering, heat a frying pan with a glug of olive oil on a medium heat and add the meatballs. Cook until the meatballs are brown all over and cooked through. This will take around 10–15 minutes.

Divide the braised vegetables between two plates, top with the meatballs and garnish with some fresh soft herbs, like dill, or parsley, or both. Delicious served with a herby or horseradish yoghurt on the side.

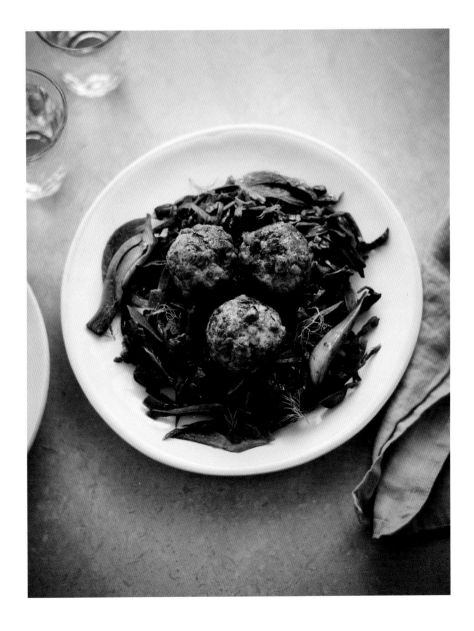

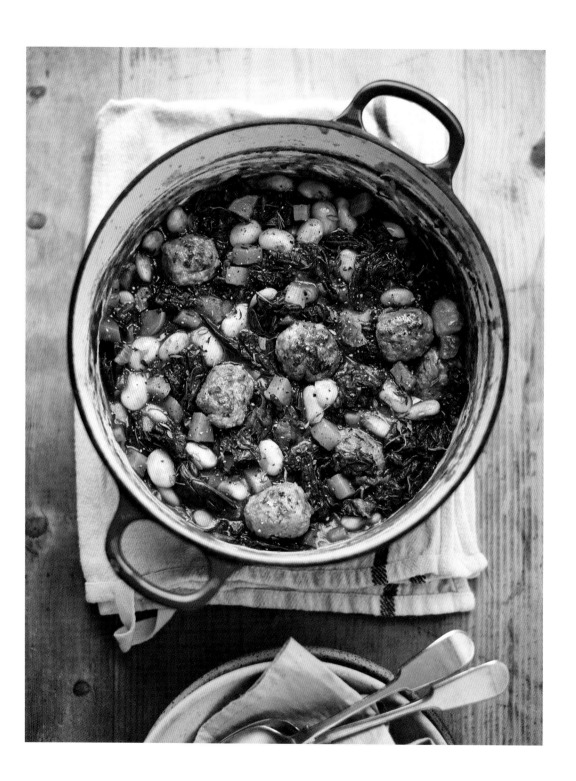

One-pan sausage and kale casserole

Serves 2

Takes 45 minutes

Hands-on: 25 minutes
Hands-off: 20 minutes

4 sausages, high pork content (around 90% or more is ideal)

400g tin of butter beans, drained and rinsed

2 tablespoons olive oil

1 onion, peeled and diced

2 carrots, peeled and diced

3 cloves of garlic, peeled and finely grated

1 sprig of rosemary, finely chopped

1 tablespoon thyme leaves

1 tablespoon arrowroot powder

400g tin of chopped tomatoes

300ml vegetable stock (you can use homemade stock (page 258) or shop-bought fresh stock is also a good option if you can't find a stock cube with straightforward-sounding ingredients)

200g kale, tough stalks removed, leaves roughly chopped

salt and black pepper

Sausages and hearty butter beans enveloped in a rich, herby tomato sauce with a generous helping of kale stirred through — this is one pan full of a whole lot of tasty goodness.

Remove the sausage meat from its casing, roll into 3 balls per sausage, and set to one side.

Tip the butter beans into a sieve or colander set over the sink, then rinse under a running cold tap until the water runs clear, which usually takes about 30 seconds.

Heat the olive oil in a casserole pot and add the onion, carrot and garlic. Cook gently for around 10 minutes, until softened and just starting to turn golden brown. Remove the veg from the pan to a plate and set to one side.

Add the herbs and the sausagemeat balls to the pan that you cooked the veg in. Add a splash more olive oil if needed and cook until the sausage is browned all over.

Return the veg to the pan, sprinkle over the arrowroot and stir to combine it with everything in the pan. Add the butter beans, tomatoes and stock. Mix it all together and bring to a simmer, then leave to bubble away and thicken up for 15–20 minutes.

Add the kale leaves and cook for another 5 minutes.

Season with salt and pepper, and serve.

Fantastic noodles

Serves 2

Takes 15 minutes

The name says it all, these fiery, flavoursome noodles are fantastic. Ideal for using up leftover veg or chicken – add more chilli if you like things hot and more prawns and chicken if you have extra available.

2 tablespoons olive oil

1 red pepper, deseeded and thinly sliced

1 bunch of spring onions, sliced

2 cloves of garlic, peeled and finely grated

2cm piece of ginger, peeled and grated

2 teaspoons mild curry powder

1 teaspoon ground turmeric

½ teaspoon chilli powder

1 egg, lightly beaten

2 large courgettes, spiralized (or you can buy packets of spiralized courgettes from the supermarket vegetable chiller, ingredients: courgettes)

100g roast chicken, shredded (ideal for using up leftovers, or you can use roast chicken from the deli section – if you do, make sure it has only one ingredient – chicken!)

100g prawns, cooked

100g beansprouts

1 tablespoon sesame oil

To serve

fresh chilli, sliced

1 tablespoon roughly chopped coriander leaves

soy sauce (check ingredients – soy-beans, salt and water only is best)

Heat the olive oil in a large wok or frying pan on a high heat. When hot, add the pepper and spring onions and cook for 2–3 minutes, until just starting to soften. Add the garlic and ginger and toss to combine, then add the spices and cook for a further 2–3 minutes.

Move everything to one side of the pan and add the egg. Quickly scramble it by moving it briskly in the pan with a wooden spoon or spatula, then stir into the veg and add the courgettes, chicken, prawns, beansprouts and sesame oil. Keep everything moving by tossing the pan.

Cook for 1–2 minutes, until the courgette noodles just start to soften, and the chicken and prawns are hot through. You don't want to over-cook the courgette noodles or they will become very watery.

Serve immediately, with some fresh chilli and coriander leaves, and splash over some soy sauce if you like.

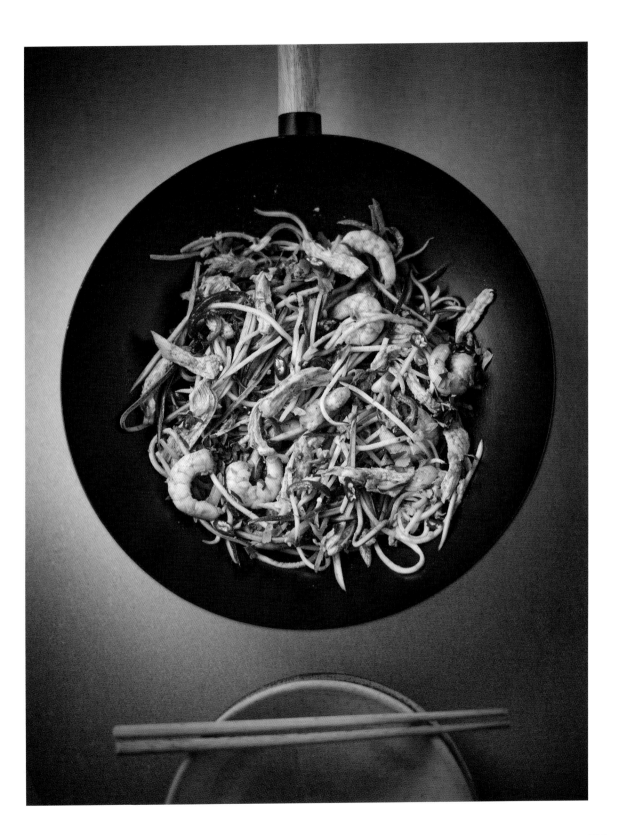

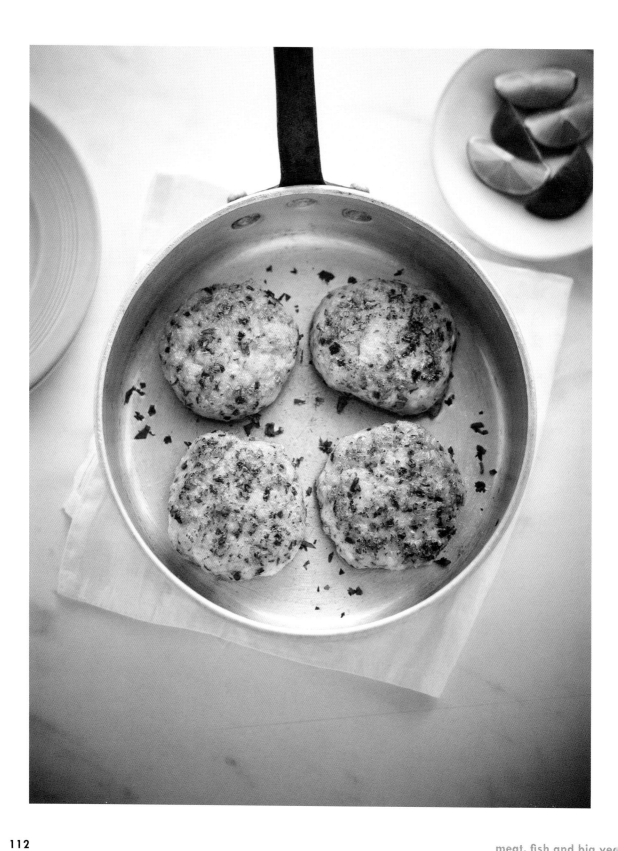

meat, fish and big veg

Prawn fishcakes

Serves 2

Takes 25 minutes

300g raw king prawns (fresh, or frozen and defrosted)

150g cod fillet (fresh, or frozen and defrosted)

2 tablespoons finely chopped coriander

1 stalk of lemongrass, tough outer layers removed, inside finely chopped

1 red chilli, deseeded and finely chopped

1 unwaxed lime, zest only

1 tablespoon olive oil

To serve

finely chopped coriander

lime wedges

These aromatic fishcakes with their crunchy golden crumb, citrus zing and chilli heat are packed full of fresh flavours. Delicious served on a bed of greens with a final twist of lime and a sprinkle of fragrant fresh coriander.

If using frozen prawns, and/or frozen cod fillet, defrost according to the packet instructions. Place the prawns and cod in a mini chopper or food processor and blitz to a paste. Add the remaining ingredients, apart from the olive oil, and pulse to just combine.

Dampen your hands and divide the mix into 2 larger or 4 smaller patties.

Heat the olive oil and fry the patties on a medium heat for 6–7 minutes, then flip and cook the other side. As the fishcakes are cooking, press down on them gently to help remove a little excess moisture.

Transfer to a plate and sprinkle over some more chopped coriander.

Serve piping hot, with a lime wedge, on a bed of green veg such as steamed spinach or alongside a green leaf salad.

One-pan prawn and chorizo skillet

Serves 2

Takes 25 minutes

1 tablespoon olive oil

100g cooking chorizo, peeled and cut into bite-size chunks

1 onion, peeled and cut into chunks

1 red or green pepper, deseeded and cut into chunks

1 courgette, cut into chunks

300g raw king prawns (fresh, or frozen and defrosted)

1 teaspoon Cajun spice mix (check that it's sugar-free)

1 tablespoon chopped parsley

salt and pepper

To serve

2 tablespoons sour cream

1 jalapeño chilli, sliced

lemon wedges

Salty, meaty chorizo is always a perfect foil to the delicate flavour of king prawns. Fire them up with the Cajun spice mix and jalapeño, then cool right down with a tangy side of sour cream. Delicious served with Tenderstem broccoli and sugar snap peas.

If using frozen prawns, defrost according to the packet instructions.

Heat the oil in a heavy-bottomed frying pan or skillet, on a high heat, and add the chorizo. Cook for 5 minutes, until the chorizo has started to go brown and release some of its fat.

Add the onion, pepper and courgette and cook for another 8 minutes, until everything is golden and starting to soften.

Add the prawns and Cajun spice mix, season with salt and pepper, and cook for 2–3 minutes, until the prawns are cooked through. Add the parsley and toss to mix.

Divide between two plates and top with sour cream, slices of jalapeño, and some lemon wedges for extra citrus freshness.

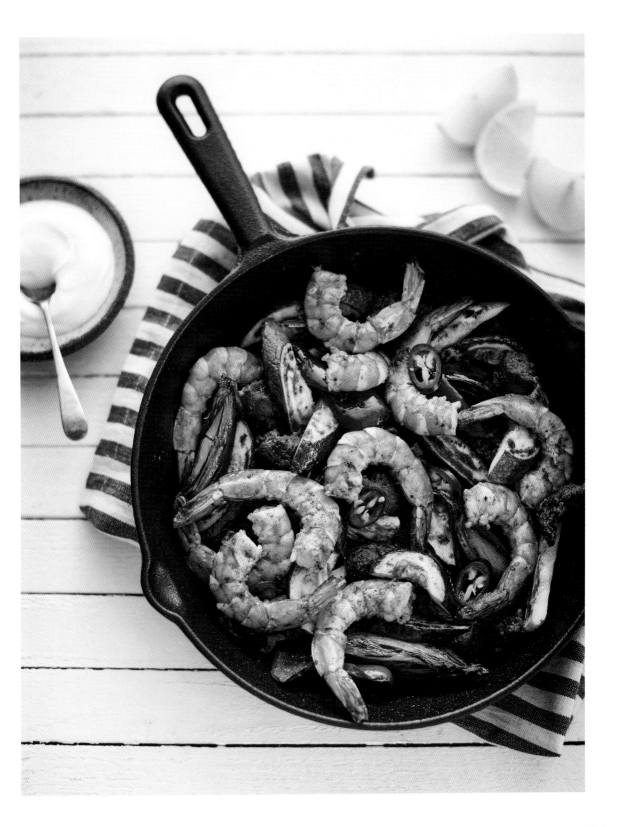

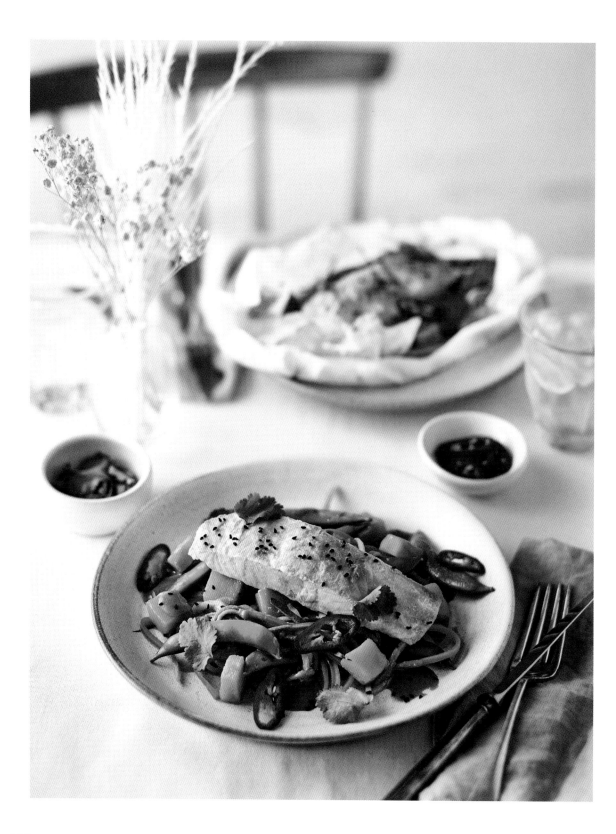

Salmon rainbow parcels

Serves 2

Takes 20 minutes

2 courgettes, peeled into ribbons or spiralized (or you can buy packets of spiralized courgettes from the supermarket vegetable chiller, ingredients: courgettes)

½ butternut squash

2 carrots, spiralized or grated

100g sugar snap peas

2 skinless, boneless salmon fillets (approx. 150g each) (fresh, or frozen and defrosted)

For the sauce

1 tablespoon white miso

1 tablespoon soy sauce (check ingredients – soybeans, salt and water only is best)

2cm piece of ginger, peeled and grated

2 cloves of garlic, peeled and grated

3 tablespoons water (approx.)

To serve

1 red chilli, sliced (leave the seeds in if you like the heat)

coriander leaves

nigella seeds

This delicious salmon is infused with fresh umami flavours and packaged up with layers of vegetable goodness – these quick colourful parcels are a sure-fire special delivery.

If using frozen salmon, defrost according to the packet instructions.

Preheat the oven to 200°C/180°C fan/gas 6.

Take two large pieces of baking paper or foil and just off-centre place half the veg on each. Top each pile of veg with a salmon fillet.

Mix together the miso, soy, ginger, garlic and as much of the water as needed to make a pouring sauce.

Drizzle the sauce over the fish and veg, then carefully fold over the paper or foil and turn up the edge all around to make a parcel. Slide on to a baking tray and repeat with the other parcel.

Place the tray in the oven for 12–15 minutes.

Be careful on opening the parcel, as there can be a lot of steam. Gently slide the contents on to a serving plate and top with some fresh red chilli, coriander leaves and nigella seeds.

Roast salmon with beetroot and lentils

Serves 2

Takes 45 minutes

Hands-on: 20 minutes
Hands-off: 25 minutes

2 salmon fillets (approx. 180g each), skin on (fresh, or frozen and defrosted)

400g tin of brown lentils, drained and rinsed

2 tablespoons olive oil

1 red onion, peeled and finely diced

2 beetroots, peeled and grated

2 teaspoons wholegrain mustard

2 tablespoons crème fraîche

2 tablespoons chopped fresh dill

40g rocket leaves

salt and black pepper

To serve

lemon wedges

Roasted, blush pink salmon on a bed of creamy, sweet beetroot and earthy lentils makes this a glorious and filling meal. Packed with fibre-rich lentils loved by your gut bacteria as well as lots of fish-oil goodness means that this delicious dish also happens to have health benefits too! The perfect combination.

If using frozen salmon, defrost according to the packet instructions.

Preheat the oven to 220°C/200°C fan/gas 7 and line a small roasting tin with baking paper. Place the salmon fillets in the roasting tin, season with black pepper, then roast in the oven for around 12–15 minutes. Once done, the flesh of the salmon should flake and separate easily along the white lines that run across the fillet when gently pressed down with a fork.

While the salmon is in the oven, tip the lentils into a sieve or colander set over the sink and rinse under the cold tap for about 30 seconds until the water draining off runs clear.

Heat the olive oil in a sauté pan or frying pan on a medium heat and add the onion. Cook for 5 minutes, until just starting to soften, then add the beets. Cook for around 8–10 minutes, until the beetroot softens. Add the lentils and cook for a minute or two. Add the mustard, crème fraîche and a splash of water, and cook until the sauce starts to thicken. Stir in the dill and some seasoning.

Remove from the heat and add the rocket. Stir through quickly and divide between two serving plates. Top each plate with a salmon fillet and a lemon wedge. This would also go well with a side of rocket salad or some steamed broccoli.

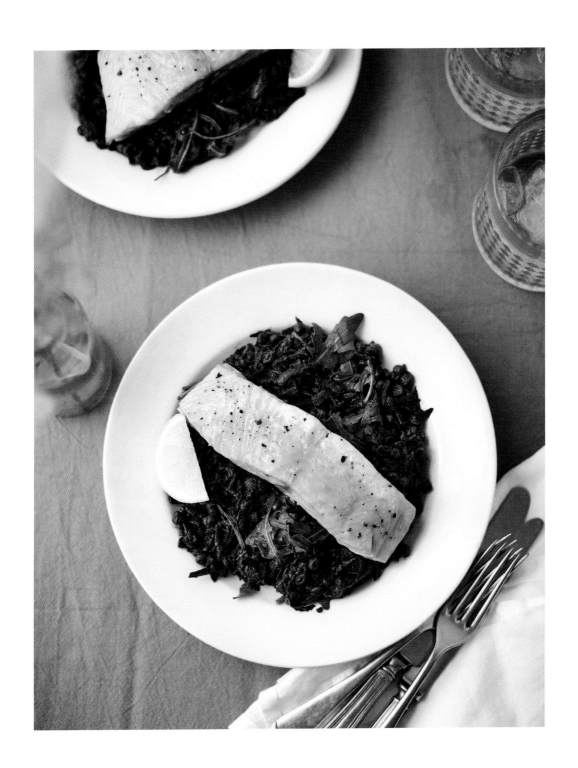

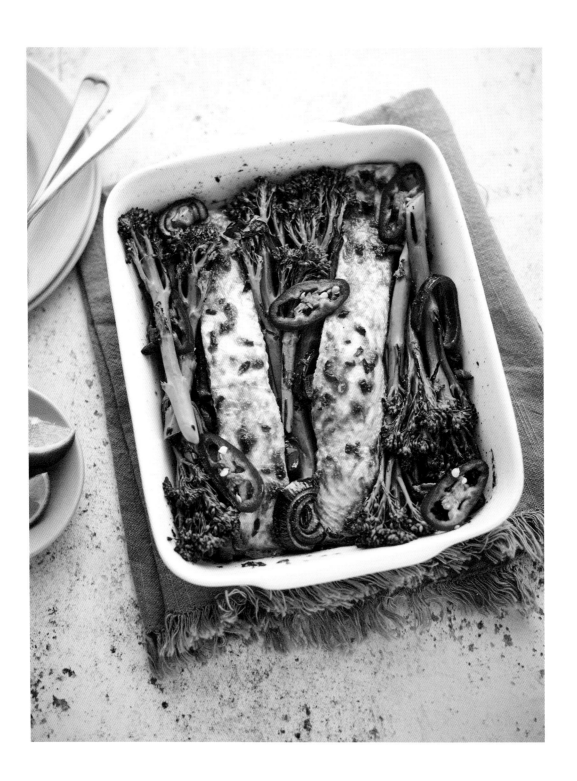

Fiery salmon and broccoli traybake

Serves 2

Takes 25 minutes, plus minimum of 1 hour to marinate

2 salmon fillets (approx. 150g each), skinless and boneless (fresh, or frozen and defrosted)

For the marinade

2 tablespoons sesame oil

1 tablespoon rice vinegar

1 tablespoon soy sauce (ideal ingredients are water, soybeans and salt)

2 cloves of garlic, peeled and grated

3cm ginger, peeled and grated

2 red chillies, chopped (leave the seeds in if you like the heat)

To bake the salmon

1 red onion, peeled and sliced into eight, layers separated

200g Tenderstem broccoli

1 tablespoon olive oil

To serve

1 lime, halved

This simple traybake packs in a lot of flavour – the magic here is that the longer you leave the salmon to infuse, the better this dish tastes. Delicious served warm from the oven, this is also super-tasty as leftovers, eaten cold or flaked into a green leaf salad.

If using frozen salmon, defrost according to the packet instructions.

Place the salmon fillets in a small shallow dish.

Put the sesame oil, vinegar, soy sauce, garlic, ginger and the chopped chillies into a small bowl, mix well, then pour over the salmon. Cover the bowl and place in the fridge to marinate for at least an hour, but if you can leave it overnight the flavour will be even better.

Preheat the oven to 200°C/180°C fan/gas 6.

Line a roasting tin with baking paper and add the salmon fillets, the onion slices and the Tenderstem broccoli. Drizzle over the marinade and a little olive oil.

Roast in the oven for 20 minutes, until the edges of the salmon have started to caramelize and the broccoli is al dente.

Serve each salmon fillet alongside half the vegetables, with a lime wedge.

Almond and herb crusted salmon fillets with steamed greens

Serves 2

Takes 30 minutes

2 salmon fillets (approx. 200g each), skin on (fresh, or frozen and defrosted)

2 teaspoons olive oil

30g almonds

1 tablespoon roughly chopped parsley

1 tablespoon roughly chopped chives

1 spring onion, roughly chopped

½ teaspoon chilli powder

1 egg white, lightly beaten

¼ teaspoon nigella seeds

250g mixed leafy greens (such as spring greens, cavolo nero, kale), sliced

10g butter

salt and black pepper

This salmon topped with aromatic fresh herbs and sweet crunchy almonds is deliciously good and just perfect served on a bed of hot buttered greens.

If using frozen salmon, defrost according to the packet instructions.

Preheat the oven to 220°C/200°C fan/gas 7 and line a small roasting tin with baking paper.

Place the salmon fillets in the roasting tin, skin side down, and pat dry with a piece of kitchen paper, then coat each fillet with a teaspoon of olive oil.

Put the almonds, parsley, chives, spring onion and chilli powder into a mini chopper or the small bowl of a food processor and blitz to a crumbly paste.

Transfer to a mixing bowl and add just enough beaten egg white to bring it together, without making it wet. Stir in the nigella seeds.

Divide the mix between the 2 salmon fillets, to cover the top of the fish.

Place the roasting tin in the hot oven and cook for 10–12 minutes, until the top of the salmon is golden brown.

While the fish is roasting, place the greens in a steamer basket and cook over simmering water for 4–5 minutes, until al dente. Drain away the steaming water and put the greens back into the pan with the butter and some seasoning. Toss until the butter has melted and the greens are coated.

Divide the greens between two serving plates and top each with a crusted salmon fillet.

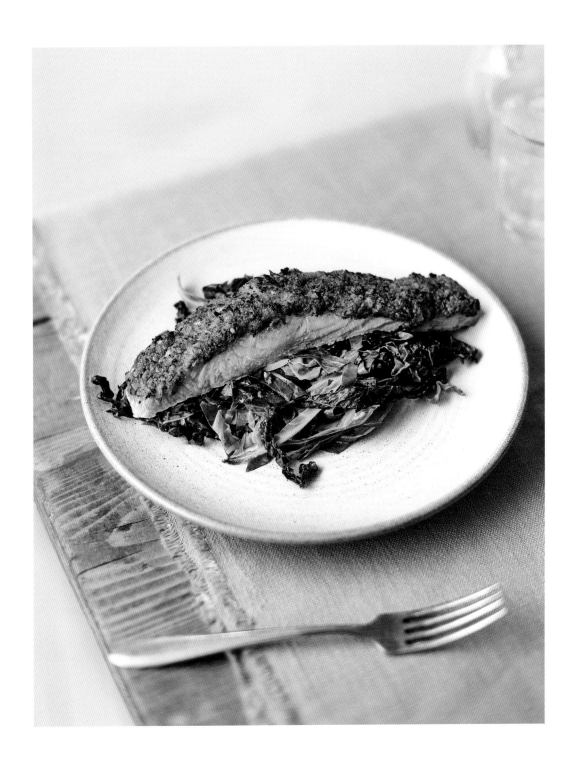

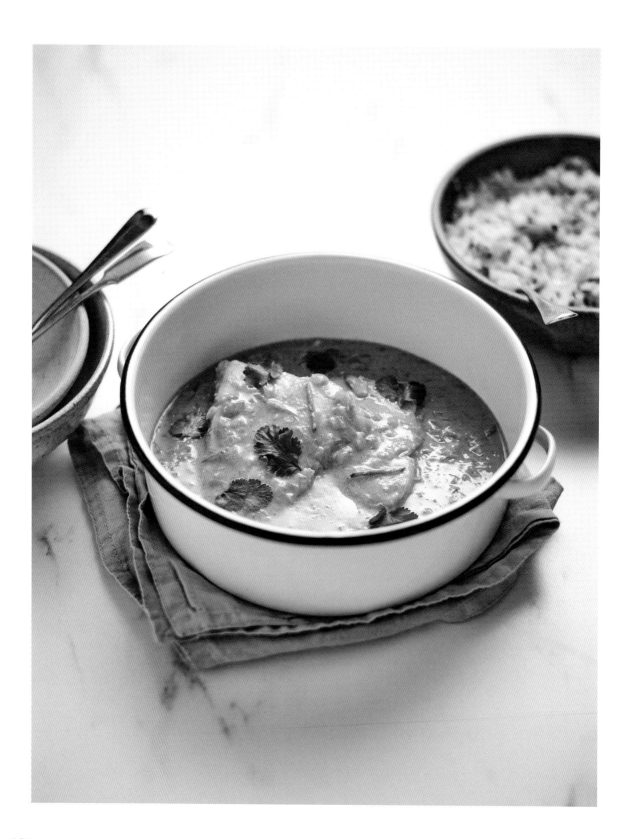

Coconut fish curry

Serves 2

Takes 30 minutes

Delicate white fish enveloped in sweet, creamy coconut, infused with spices and fresh herbs – this velvety warming curry is a feast for all your senses.

400ml coconut milk, made from creamed coconut (roughly 100g)

1 tablespoon olive oil

1 onion, diced

1 stalk of lemongrass, tough outer layers removed, inside very finely chopped

2 cloves of garlic, peeled and finely grated

3cm piece of fresh ginger, peeled and finely grated

1 teaspoon ground coriander

½ teaspoon ground turmeric

½ teaspoon ground cumin

2 lime leaves

1 tablespoon desiccated coconut

2 x 150g white fish fillets, such as cod, hake or pollack (fresh or frozen and defrosted)

To serve

coriander leaves

If using frozen fish fillets, defrost according to the packet instructions.

Chop the creamed coconut into pieces and place in a saucepan. Cover with 400ml of boiling water and heat gently, stirring for around 10 minutes until the pieces have dissolved.

Heat the olive oil in a casserole dish and add the onion, lemongrass, garlic and ginger. Cook on a medium heat for around 10 minutes, until everything has softened, but without it catching much colour.

Add the spices and lime leaves, and stir well to combine. Add the desiccated coconut and the creamed coconut mixture and cook for 10 minutes to reduce slightly.

Add the fish and cook for 7–8 minutes, until cooked through.

Serve with steamed greens (such as broccoli and spring greens), or on a bed of cauliflower rice (page 216).

Top with coriander leaves.

Harissa cod with roasted veg and lentils

Serves 6

Takes 55 minutes

Hands-on: 5 minutes
Hands-off: 50 minutes

6 x 160g skinless, boneless
cod fillets (fresh, or frozen
and defrosted)

2 tablespoons harissa paste
(no added sugar)

salt

For the veg

2 x 400g tins of Puy lentils,
drained and rinsed

4 peppers, mixed colours,
deseeded and cut into
chunks

200g Tenderstem broccoli

2 courgettes, cut into chunks

6 ripe tomatoes, quartered

3 tablespoons olive oil

150ml vegetable stock
(homemade (page 259) or a
shop-bought fresh stock if you
can't find a stock cube with
straightforward ingredients)

salt and black pepper

To serve

100g full-fat Greek yoghurt

1 unwaxed lime, zest only

2 tablespoons finely chopped
coriander leaves

Harissa is a fiery chilli paste alive with garlic and smoked spices. A versatile storecupboard go-to, it's also delicious rubbed on to sizzling grilled lamb or mixed into a kaleidoscope of roasted veggies.

If using frozen cod fillets, defrost according to the packet instructions.

Preheat the oven to 200°C/180°C fan/gas 6.

Season the fish with a pinch of salt, then rub the harissa paste all over the fish fillets and set to one side.

Tip the lentils into a sieve or colander set over the sink and rinse under a running cold tap for about 30 seconds, until the water runs off clear.

Place the vegetables in a large roasting tin, add the olive oil, season with salt and pepper and toss everything to coat with the oil and seasoning.

Roast the vegetables in the oven for 40 minutes, turning halfway by removing the baking tray from the oven and giving everything a big stir before putting it back into the oven for the rest of the cooking time.

Remove from the oven, add the lentils and the stock, and stir. Lay the harissa cod on top. Return to the oven for another 8–10 minutes, until the fish is just cooked through – if you press it gently, the fish should flake apart.

Remove the roasting tin from the oven. Plate up and add generous dollops of thick Greek yoghurt around the edge. Grate over the lime zest and scatter over the fresh coriander leaves before serving.

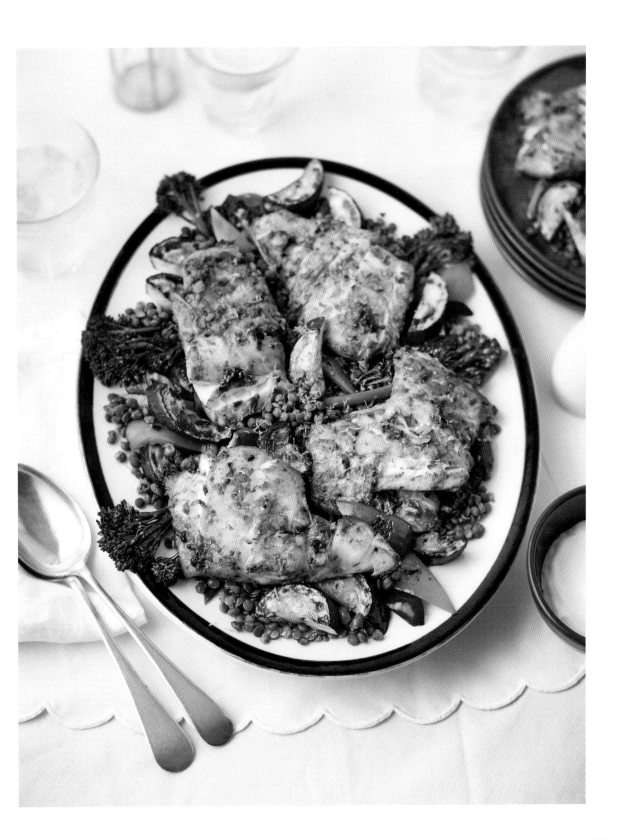

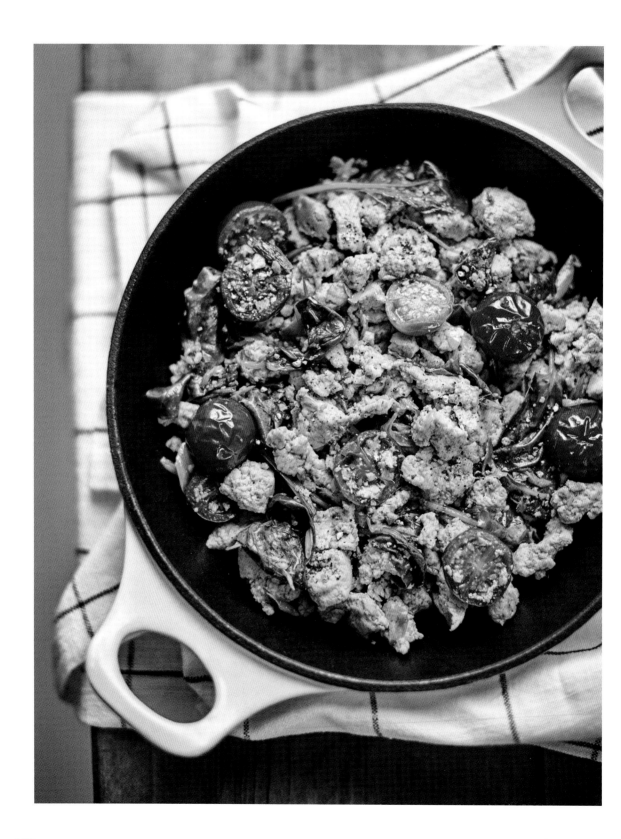

meat, fish and big ve

Spiced tofu scramble

  Vegan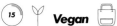

Serves 2

Takes 10 minutes

15g butter, or 1 tablespoon olive oil

1 bunch of spring onions, chopped

280g firm tofu

12 cherry tomatoes, halved

½ teaspoon garam masala

¼ teaspoon ground turmeric

40g spinach leaves

black pepper

squeeze of lime juice

It's a Full Diet joy that a dish this quick and easy can be so full of flavour. Add more of the spices depending on your taste preference, and if you'd like to make this a vegan meal, choose a plant-based fat such as olive oil.

Heat the butter or olive oil in a frying pan over a medium heat and add the spring onions. Cook for a minute or two until just softening.

While the spring onions are cooking, crumble the tofu using either your hands or a fork or potato masher. Add the tofu to the pan containing the spring onions along with the tomatoes, garam masala and turmeric.

Cook all together for a few minutes, combining everything and allowing any water in the tofu to evaporate and the tomatoes to start to break down.

Add the spinach leaves and a good twist of black pepper. Stir gently until just wilted. Finally add a squeeze of lime juice, then serve immediately.

Five-spice tofu lettuce wraps

 Vegan

Serves 2

Takes 20 minutes,
plus pressing time

250g block of firm tofu

1 tablespoon Chinese
five-spice

1 tablespoon sesame oil

1 carrot, julienned (cut into
long thin batons)

100g white cabbage,
shredded

100g sugar snaps, sliced into
thirds

1 tablespoon toasted sesame
seeds (black or white)

salt and black pepper

For the dressing

1 tablespoon soy sauce
(check ingredients – ideally
these should be water,
soybeans and salt)

2 teaspoons ponzu (make
sure there's no added sugar),
or alternatively freshly
squeezed lemon juice

To serve

2 cos lettuces, base trimmed
and leaves pulled apart

fresh coriander, chopped

sliced red chillies (optional)

Crispy tofu, coated with a heady mix of fragrant spices and wrapped in a fresh crisp lettuce leaf. Gorgeously tasty finger food at its best.

First press as much water out of the tofu as possible, to give you a perfect crunch when cooked. Lay the tofu between sheets of kitchen paper, and place something heavy on the top sheet, pressing it for at least half an hour, changing the paper as needed when it becomes wet.

Once the tofu is ready, cut it into 1.5cm cubes. Put the cubes into a bowl and add the five-spice and some seasoning. Toss everything together until coated, then put to one side.

Heat the oil in a wok, sauté pan or frying pan and add the tofu. Cook on a high heat for around 6–8 minutes, tossing and shaking the pan to keep the tofu moving. Once golden brown, remove to a plate and add all the vegetables to the same pan. Cook the veg for 1–2 minutes, then add the tofu and sesame seeds and stir well to mix.

Next, mix a simple dressing of soy and ponzu (or freshly squeezed lemon juice).

To make the wraps, arrange the lettuce leaves in a row and work your way along, filling them with the tofu-veg mixture. Drizzle over the dressing, garnish with fresh corriander and sliced chilli (if using), then pick up and enjoy!

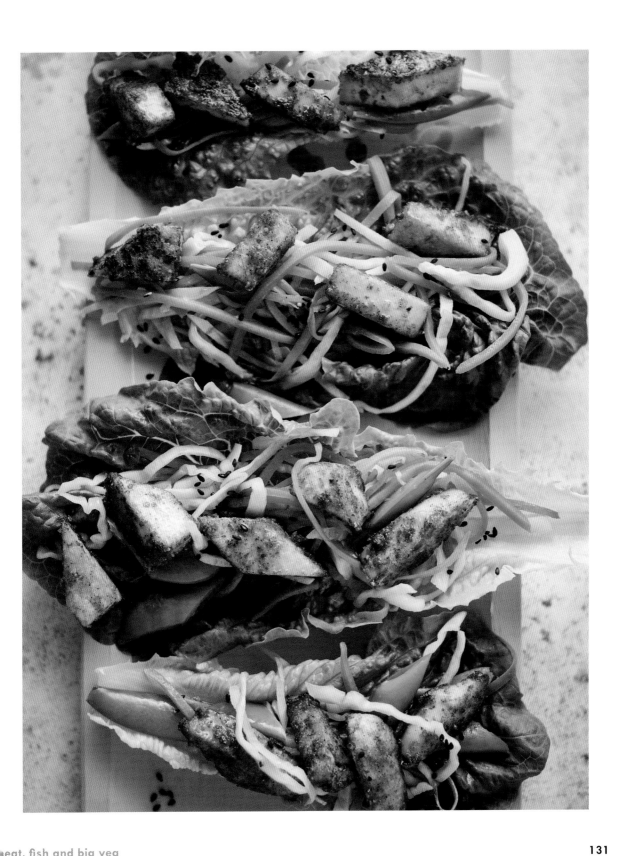

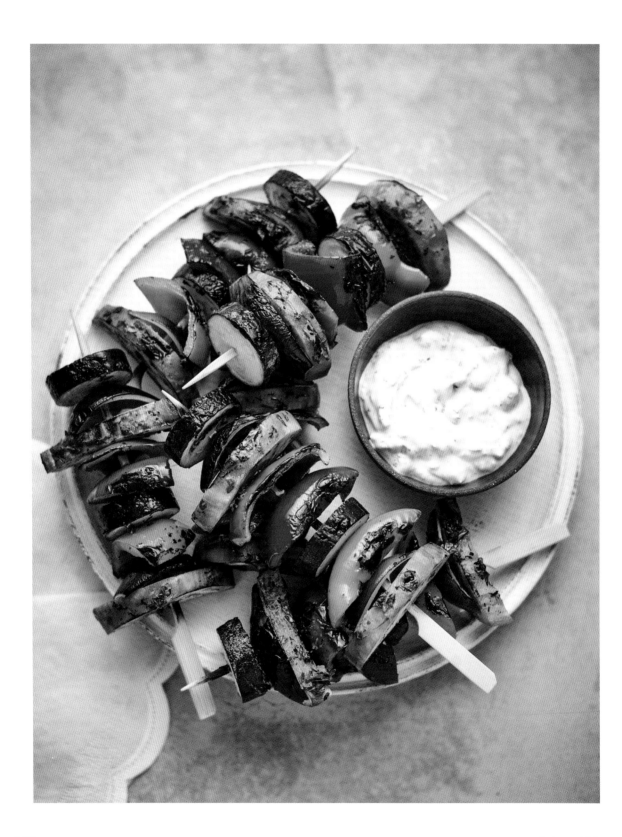

Veggie kebabs

 Vegan

Serves 2

Takes 25 minutes

1 courgette, sliced into 5mm rounds

1 red pepper, deseeded and cut into chunks

1 yellow pepper, deseeded and cut into chunks

1 green pepper, deseeded and cut into chunks

1 aubergine, peeled and cut into chunks

1 red onion, peeled and cut into quarters, layers separated

For the marinade

3 tablespoons olive oil

1 tablespoon finely chopped parsley

1 clove of garlic, finely grated

To serve (optional)

hummus

tzatziki

olive oil

crunchy sea salt crystals.

Full of phytonutrient goodness that is loved by your gut bacteria – if there was ever a perfect example of eating a rainbow then this is it! These kebabs taste as good as they look, and they work really well on a barbecue too.

Put all the ingredients for the marinade into a large bowl and mix well. Add the vegetables and toss to coat.

Take 4 long skewers and divide the vegetables between them, alternating the colours to create a beautiful rainbow effect. Reserve any leftover marinade.

If you are using wooden skewers, to ensure they don't catch fire in the grill or barbecue, cover any exposed wood with foil or, alternatively, soak the skewers in water for 5 minutes before using.

Take a grill pan and lay the kebabs on the metal grill pan tracks.

Heat your grill to the hottest setting, and once hot place the kebabs under the grill until you start to see some colour developing, then turn, basting the kebabs with the leftover marinade.

Repeat for all four sides, adding more marinade as you go.

Cook for around 20 minutes in total, or until the veg are cooked to your liking.

Serve straight away, or cool and add to your lunchbox or salad. Great dipped into hummus or tzatziki, or simply served with a drizzle of olive oil and a sprinkle of crunchy sea salt crystals.

Cauliflower crust pizza

Serves 2

Takes 1 hour 20 minutes

Hands-on: 35 minutes
Hands-off: 45 minutes

1 extra large cauliflower

150g feta, crumbled

2 tablespoons ground
flaxseed

1 tablespoon dried oregano

black pepper

Topping per pizza

1 tablespoon tomato purée

75g mozzarella, torn

plus your choice of ham,
mushrooms, olives, peppers,
chicken, wilted spinach, chilli,
egg (cracked on top before
baking, Florentine style),
mixed cheese, tomato,
chorizo, chilli flakes, basil
leaves and any other pizza
topping you like!

The crisp cauliflower base makes this just about the only pizza your gut bacteria love too! Enjoy the tangy tomato and bubbling mozzarella and choose from a finery of toppings – pile on what you have in, experiment and make it up to embrace this deliciously versatile Programme classic as your own.

Preheat the oven to 190°C/170°C fan/gas 5.

Cut the cauliflower into florets, and discard the stalk. Place the florets in the bowl of a food processor and blitz to a rice-like consistency. Alternatively, you can grate the florets on a box grater.

Once you have the cauliflower turned into rice, put it into a large non-stick frying pan or wok. Stirring fairly constantly, cook it for 10–15 minutes on a medium heat until it has lost around a third of its bulk and is dried out. Lay out a clean tea towel and pour the cooked cauliflower into the middle, then gather up the corners and wring it out over the sink. This will remove any excess moisture out of the cauliflower and ensure the pizza base crisps up nicely.

Put the cauliflower rice into a large mixing bowl along with the feta, flaxseed, oregano and some black pepper. Mix everything together well with your hands, so that the mix sticks together.

Divide the mix into two equal amounts and get two large pieces of non-stick baking paper ready. Shape the cauliflower into two pizza rounds, one on each piece of baking paper. Use a rolling pin to help keep an even thickness.

Keeping the pizza bases on the baking paper, carefully slide them on to a baking tray, then put into the oven for 25–30 minutes, checking occasionally that they are cooking evenly and aren't burning on the edges. You might need to turn the trays around occasionally.

Remove from the oven, turn the heat down to 170°C/150°C fan/gas 3 and carefully turn the bases over. Pop them back into the oven for another 10 minutes. The base should be really dried out now.

Remove from the oven, and now it's time to build your pizza. Spread over the tomato purée, then add some mozzarella and your choice of toppings. Bake for another 5–6 minutes, until the cheese has melted and is bubbling and your toppings have taken on a bit of colour. Eat immediately.

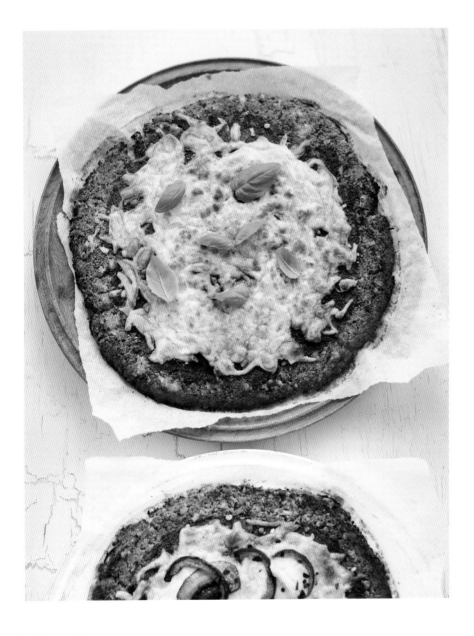

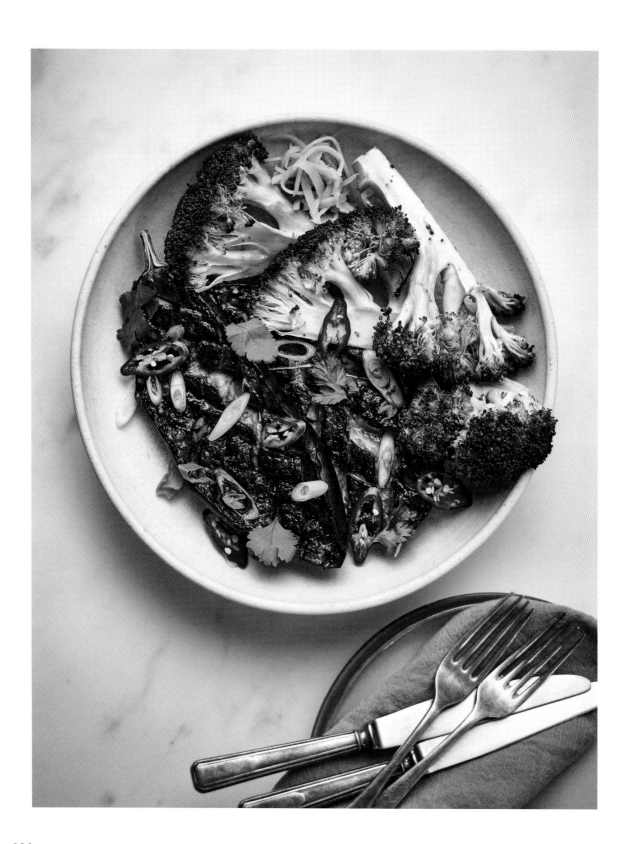

Miso roasted aubergines and broccoli

 Vegan

Serves 2

Takes 45 minutes

Treat your gut bacteria to a feast with this probiotic-rich miso. A contrast of flavours – the salty soy sauce sets off the sweetness of the mirin, all cut through by the broccoli's fresh green crunch. Delicious eaten at home, it also travels well for a delicious meal on the go.

1 large aubergine

60g red miso

1 tablespoon sesame oil

2 teaspoons soy sauce

1–2 teaspoons mirin

2 teaspoons rice vinegar

For the broccoli

½ head of broccoli, cut in half, then into quarters, through the stalk

1 tablespoon sesame oil

To serve

4 spring onions, sliced

1 red chilli, sliced

pickled ginger (optional, to taste)

coriander leaves

Preheat the oven to 190°C/170°C fan/gas 5 and line a roasting tin with baking paper.

Cut the aubergine in half lengthways and then carefully, without going through the skin, score a diamond pattern in the flesh. Place the aubergine halves in the roasting tin, skin side down.

Mix together the miso, sesame oil, soy sauce, mirin and rice vinegar. Put roughly a quarter of the mix on each aubergine half and spread over to coat all the flesh. Roast in the oven for 30 minutes.

Remove from the oven and add the rest of the sauce. It should now get into some of the criss-crosses as the aubergines soften.

Add the broccoli to the tray, then drizzle the sesame oil over everything.

Return the tray to the oven for another 15 minutes. The flesh of the aubergine should be very soft and tender and on the verge of collapse. If there is any resistance, return the tray to the oven for another 5–10 minutes.

When the aubergines are done, remove them from the tray and serve one half each, alongside half the broccoli. Scatter over the spring onions, red chilli, pickled ginger and coriander leaves.

Halloumi and veg traybake

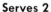

Serves 2

Takes 35 minutes

A rainbow of roasted great taste, this is about as easy as it gets. Chop, toss, roast, eat. It's that simple. And also versatile – you can sub in goat's cheese or feta for the halloumi, and if you prefer spicy rather than herby sometimes, exchange the mixed herbs for 1 teaspoon of fiery chilli flakes.

The roasted vegetables are ideal for batch cooking. When you are ready to eat them, it's at this point you cook the halloumi by adding it to the veg and heating everything up together. The roast veg also makes a great portable option – here sub in a cheese that travels well and tastes great cold, like mozzarella or feta.

1 red onion, cut into chunks

1 red pepper, deseeded and cut into chunks

1 yellow pepper, deseeded and cut into chunks

1 courgette, cut into chunks

2 tomatoes, cut into quarters

2 tablespoons extra virgin olive oil

1 tablespoon dried mixed herbs

250g halloumi, cut into 6 slices

salt and black pepper

Preheat the oven to 200°C/180°C fan/gas 6.

Put the veg into a large roasting tin and drizzle over the oil. Sprinkle over the herbs and season with salt and black pepper. Toss to coat everything, then roast in the oven for 15 minutes.

Remove the roasting tin from the oven and turn all the veg.

Add the halloumi slices, nestling them in among the veg, then return the tin to the oven for 12–15 minutes, until the halloumi is lightly golden.

Remove from the oven, season to taste and serve while the halloumi is piping hot.

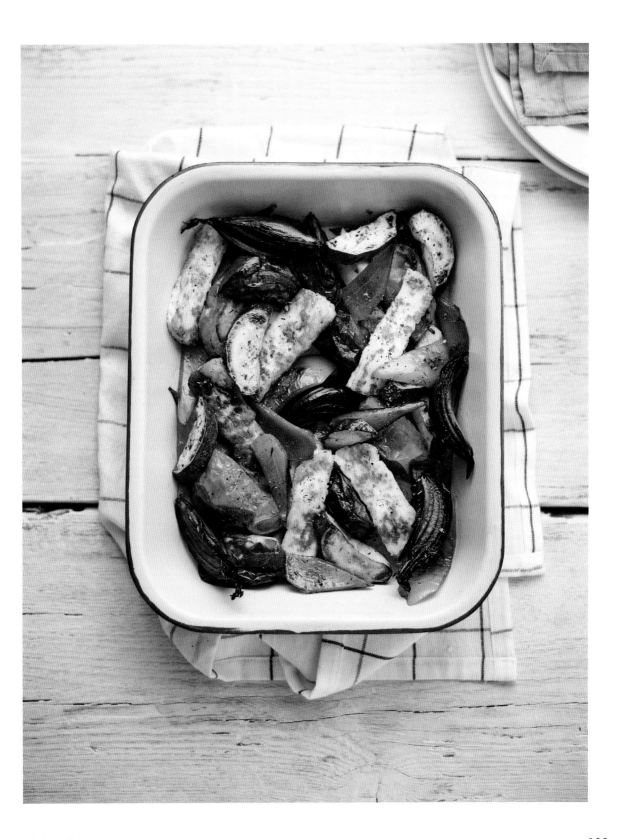

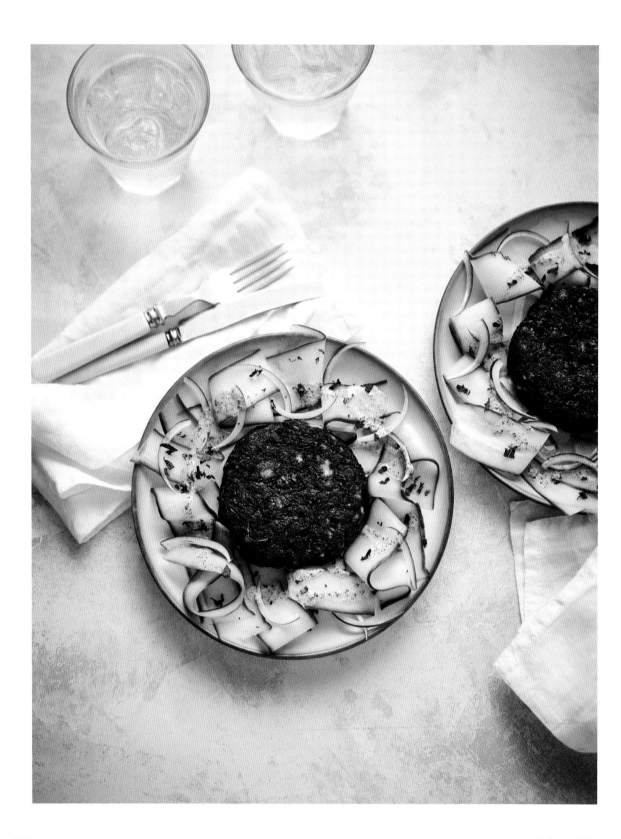

Beetroot and feta burgers with cucumber and mint salad

Serves 2

Takes 20 minutes

The sweetness of the beetroot is perfectly complemented by the salty, tangy feta and the fresh herbs. Served piping hot, the golden crunchy crumb of the burgers is just right with the cool, refreshing cucumber and mint salad. Ideal for a meal any time, and always popular served at a summer lunch party or barbecue. The burgers are also delicious eaten cold with the salad, making them an ideal portable option.

For the burgers

200g raw beetroot

100g feta, crumbled

30g ground flaxseed

1 tablespoon chopped parsley leaves

1 tablespoon chopped dill

1 unwaxed lemon, zest only

1 tablespoon olive oil

For the salad

1 small cucumber, peeled into ribbons (seeds discarded)

1 tablespoon roughly chopped mint leaves

1 small red onion, very thinly sliced (optional)

For the dressing

2 tablespoons tahini

1 lemon, juice only

1 small clove of garlic, peeled and finely grated

2 teaspoons sumac (optional)

salt and black pepper

To prepare the beetroot, grate it on a box grater, then squeeze out any excess liquid with your hands. A pair of disposable gloves is very helpful here to prevent the beetroot staining your hands.

To make the burgers, place all the ingredients except for the olive oil in a mixing bowl and use your hands to work everything together. You need to be quite firm with it to encourage it to stick and bond.

Divide the mix into two and shape each one into a burger. Heat the olive oil in a frying pan then add the burgers. Cook over a medium heat for around 6–7 minutes each side, until golden brown.

While the burgers are cooking, divide the cucumber, mint leaves and red onion (if using) between two plates.

Whisk together the dressing ingredients (or shake together in a clean jam jar), adding as much cold water as you need to get the consistency you like. Drizzle the dressing over the salad, then top with a beetroot burger.

Mushroom and lentil ragù with Parmesan

(if vegetarian
Parmesan used)

Serves 4

Takes 45 minutes

Hands-on: 25 minutes
Hands-off: 20 minutes

This rich, slow-cooked, warmly fragrant ragù luxuriously envelops the mushrooms and lentils, infusing them with its herbs and spices. Finished off with a final Parmesan flourish, this Programme favourite is always a welcome bowl of hearty flavour and goodness.

2 tablespoons olive oil

1 red onion, diced

2 sticks of celery, diced

1 carrot, peeled and diced

5 cloves of garlic, peeled and finely grated

1 tablespoon dried mixed herbs

2 teaspoons dried oregano

½ teaspoon ground or freshly grated nutmeg

2 tablespoons tomato purée

400g chestnut mushrooms, chopped

200g packet of ready-cooked Puy lentils

400g tin of chopped tomatoes

200ml vegetable stock (either homemade (page 259) or shop-bought fresh stock is also a good option if you can't find a stock cube with straightforward ingredients)

20g basil, roughly chopped

salt and black pepper

To serve

40g Parmesan, finely grated

Heat the olive oil in a large saucepan on a medium heat and add the onion, celery and carrot. Cook for 10 minutes, stirring occasionally until softened and starting to turn golden.

Add the garlic, dried herbs and nutmeg and cook for another 2 minutes. Add the tomato purée and stir into the mix.

Turn the heat up and add the mushrooms. Cook for 5–6 minutes, stirring everything together, then add the lentils, chopped tomatoes and stock.

Bring everything up to a simmer, then reduce the heat and cook until thick and sticky. This should take another 15–20 minutes.

Turn off the heat, add the basil and season to taste.

Serve on courgetti (see page 151) or on a bed of spinach leaves, which will wilt beautifully under the heat of the ragù, and top with a generous flurry of Parmesan.

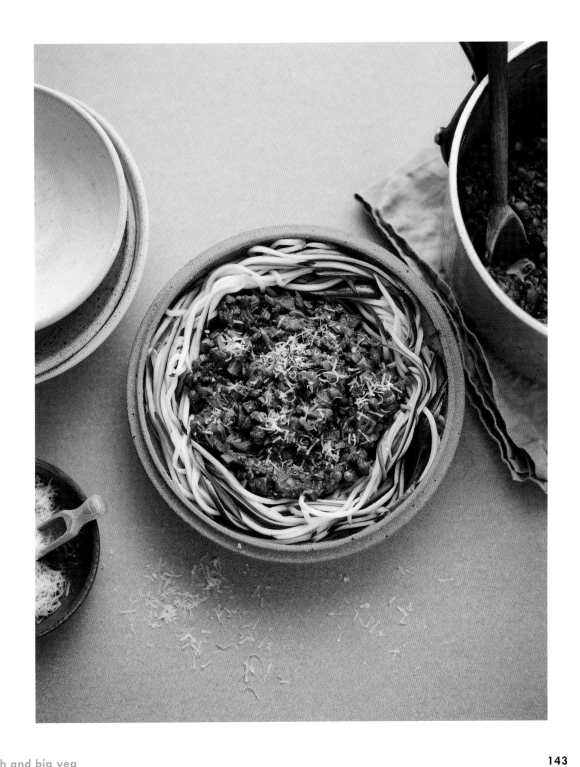

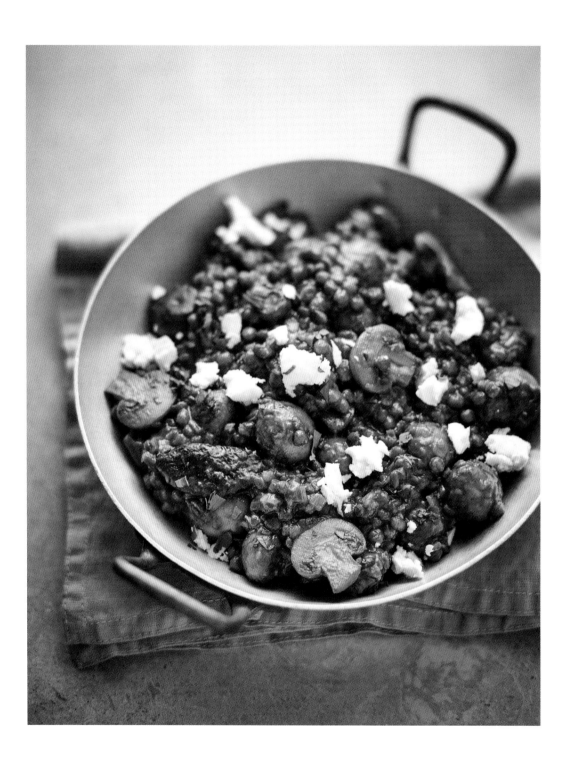

Lentils with mushrooms and goat's cheese

Serves 2

Takes 20 minutes

Dense earthy lentils, studded with buttery garlic mushrooms and tangy, creamy goat's cheese – this is a generous dish, full of rich flavours. Perfect eaten piping hot with the cheese slightly melted into the lentil base layer, or alternatively as a delicious on-the-go packed meal.

400g tin of brown lentils, drained and rinsed

30g butter

1 tablespoon olive oil

2 banana shallots, finely chopped

3 cloves of garlic, peeled and finely grated

300g mixed mushrooms (like wild, chestnut, button, shiitake or oyster)

200ml vegetable stock this can be homemade (page 259) or shop-bought fresh stock is also good here if you can't find a cube with straightforward-sounding ingredients)

1 tablespoon chopped parsley leaves

120g soft goat's cheese (usually sold as a log)

salt and black pepper

Tip the lentils into a sieve or colander set over the sink and rinse under the cold tap for about 30 seconds until the water draining out runs clear. Set to one side.

Heat the butter and oil in a large frying pan on a medium heat and add the shallots. Cook for 5 minutes, until softening without taking on much colour, then add the garlic. Cook for another 2 minutes, then turn the heat up and add the mushrooms.

Cook, tossing the mushrooms only every now and again for another 5–6 minutes. Once the mushrooms are golden, add the lentils and stock, turn the heat down and cook until the stock has almost evaporated.

Remove from the heat and stir through the parsley and some seasoning. Crumble over the goat's cheese and serve.

Aubergine, tomato and pine nut roast

 Vegan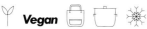

Serves 2

Takes 1 hour

Hands-on: 15 minutes
Hands-off: 45–50 minutes

This richly spiced nut roast makes for hearty, plant-based eating. Roasted aubergines are a versatile base for a host of fillings – a bit like a jacket potato without the associated blood sugar rise. For variety you can also roast the aubergines according to the base recipe and then load them up with cheese, herbs and garlic or any other filling you like.

2 aubergines, cut in half lengthways

olive oil (4 tablespoons for the aubergines, 2 tablespoons for cooking the onion and garlic)

1 onion, peeled and diced

4 cloves of garlic, peeled and finely grated

1 teaspoon ground coriander

½ teaspoon ground cumin

½ teaspoon ground cinnamon

½ teaspoon chilli flakes

2 tablespoons tomato purée

400g tin of chopped tomatoes

40g pine nuts

1 tablespoon chopped parsley

salt and black pepper

To serve

a handful of rocket leaves

100g full-fat Greek yoghurt (optional)

50g feta (optional)

hummus (for a vegan option)

Preheat the oven to 200°C/180°C fan/gas 6 and line a roasting tin with baking paper.

Place the aubergines snugly in the tray and use a sharp knife to score the flesh in a diamond pattern (leaving the skin intact). Use 1 tablespoon of olive oil on each aubergine half, rubbing it into the scored flesh and over the skin with your hands. Season with salt and pepper, then place the tray of aubergines in the oven and roast for 30 minutes.

While the aubergines are roasting, heat the remaining 2 tablespoons of oil in a saucepan on a medium heat and add the onion and garlic. Cook for 10 minutes, stirring often, until softened, then add the spices and tomato purée. Cook for another 5 minutes.

Add the chopped tomatoes, season with salt and pepper, stir everything together well, then allow to simmer until the aubergines have had their 30 minutes in the oven.

Remove the aubergines from the oven and top each aubergine half with the tomato mix. Scatter over the pine nuts, then return to the oven and bake for another 20–25 minutes.

Once done, remove from the oven and scatter over the parsley.

Take two plates and place a generous handful of rocket leaves on each along with two aubergine halves per person, which are delicious with some feta crumbled on top. Serve with Greek yoghurt or for a vegan option with a side of hummus.

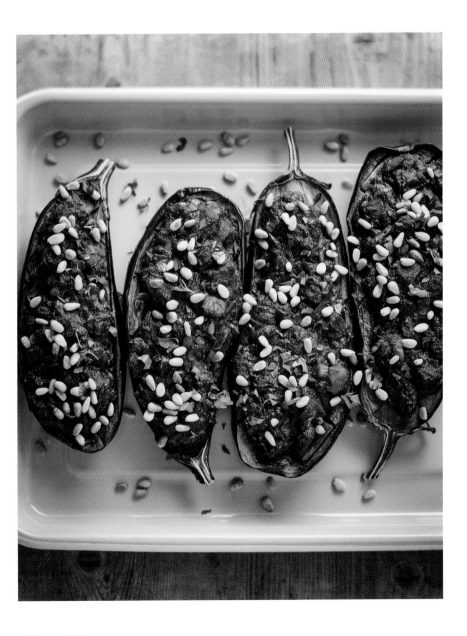

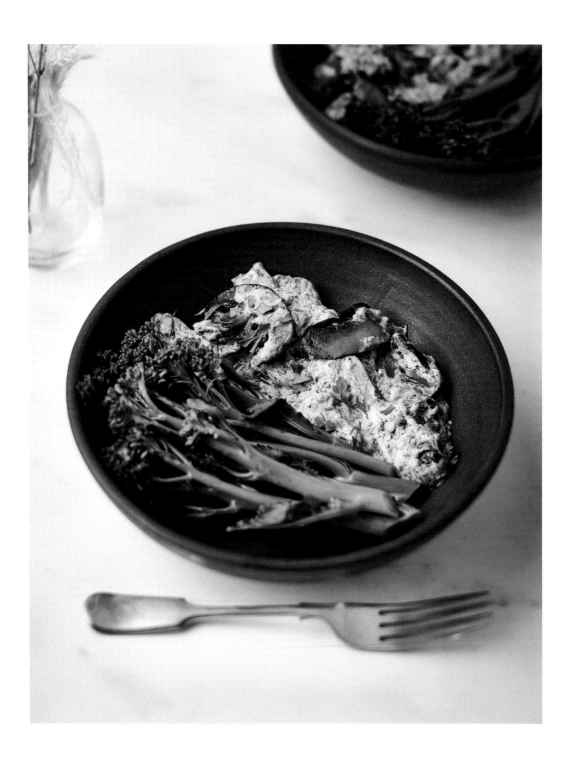

meat, fish and big v

Mushroom stroganoff

Serves 2

Takes 25 minutes

2 tablespoons olive oil

2 banana shallots, peeled and finely chopped

2 cloves of garlic, peeled and finely grated

¼ teaspoon smoked paprika

a pinch of cayenne pepper

15g butter

300g chestnut mushrooms, sliced

150ml sour cream

1 teaspoon Dijon mustard

½ lemon, juice to taste

1 tablespoon chopped parsley leaves

salt and black pepper

I have adapted a classic creamy stroganoff into a smoky, deeply flavoured plant-based version that gives the chestnut mushrooms star billing. Gorgeous served alongside fresh greens or on a bed of nutty cauliflower rice.

Heat the olive oil in a frying pan and add the shallots and garlic. Cook on a medium heat for 5 minutes, stirring, until softening, then add the paprika and cayenne pepper and cook for another minute while stirring everything together.

Remove the shallots and garlic to a dish, leaving any excess oil in the pan, and turn the heat up. Add the butter, and once foaming add the mushrooms. Cook without turning for 2 minutes, then toss all together. Don't over-stir or the mushrooms will steam and become watery – leave them to brown, then turn them and leave for another minute before turning again.

After around 5–6 minutes on a high heat, the mushrooms should be quite golden. Return the shallots and garlic to the pan and add the sour cream and mustard. Cook for a couple of minutes, stirring continuously.

Turn off the heat and add a squeeze of lemon juice, the chopped parsley and some seasoning.

Serve with steamed greens, such as broccoli or spinach, or alternatively on a bed of cauliflower rice (page 216).

Stuffed red peppers

 Vegan

Serves 4

Takes 35 minutes

4 red peppers, halved and deseeded

For the stuffing mixture

400g tin of green lentils, drained and rinsed

2 tablespoons olive oil

1 banana shallot, finely chopped

2 cloves of garlic, peeled and finely grated

2 ripe tomatoes, diced

100g feta, crumbled (leave out for a vegan option or substitute with a vegan cheese alternative)

30g walnuts, crumbled

2 teaspoons dried oregano

salt and black pepper

These treasure troves of crimson red peppers are bursting with texture and flavour. Get your eye in with this recipe and then, if you want to, you can mix and match your stuffing – for example subbing the walnuts for pine nuts or choosing a different type of cheese – mozzarella or Cheddar would also work well.

Preheat the oven to 190°C/170°C fan/gas 5.

Tip the lentils into a sieve or colander set over the sink and rinse under a running cold tap until the water runs clear, then set to one side.

Line a roasting tin with baking paper. Place the 8 pepper halves in the tin and prop them up with a little scrunched-up baking paper if needed, to keep them from rolling on to their sides.

Put all the stuffing mixture ingredients into a mixing bowl, stir well to combine, then divide between the pepper halves.

Place the roasting tin in the hot oven and cook for 25–30 minutes, until the peppers are tender and the filling is cooked through.

Serve alongside a green salad or green veg of your choosing.

Courgetti carbonara

Serves 2

Takes 10 minutes

400g courgettes (or use prepared courgetti, available from many supermarkets with one ingredient only – courgettes!)

2 eggs

50g Parmesan, grated

black pepper

80g diced pancetta

1 large clove of garlic, peeled and finely grated

To serve

extra Parmesan

a grating of fresh nutmeg

All the ham-and-eggy, cheesy goodness of a carbonara with none of the blood sugar and insulin surge of linguine. Ready almost as quickly as a ready-meal version but far more 'convenient' than anything the food industry could make for us – this carbonara is a delicious Programme classic.

Top and tail the courgettes and use a spiralizer to turn them into courgetti. Or use a vegetable peeler to peel them into ribbons for more of a pappardelle option.

Beat the 2 eggs in a bowl and add the Parmesan and some black pepper. Beat again to combine.

Bring a large pan of salted water to the boil. Place a sauté pan or frying pan on a medium high heat.

Add the courgetti to the boiling water and cook for 3 minutes. At the same time, add the pancetta and garlic to the sauté/frying pan and cook until golden. Stir often to prevent the garlic catching.

Once the pancetta is golden, use a slotted spoon to transfer the courgetti to the sauté pan along with 2 tablespoons of the courgetti cooking water. Reduce the heat to medium low.

Add the beaten egg and Parmesan mix and use a wooden spoon to stir everything together rapidly. You don't want this to catch and the egg to scramble, so keep it moving and after a minute or two you will have a deliciously glossy sauce that coats the courgetti 'pasta'.

Divide between two bowls, garnish with a sprinkle of extra Parmesan and a grating of fresh nutmeg and serve immediately.

celebration!

If in the past, you have approached eating at special occasions and get-togethers with a sense of trepidation, please feel assured that you have now found a way of eating that puts you right back in the centre of things, having fun and taking part. In many situations, your usual Programme food will work very well, for example enjoying a summer lunch party with aubergine, tomato and pine nut roast (page 146) or serving herb and garlic lamb chops (page 97) to guests at your barbecue.

At other times you might want some extra gusto, and it's here that your Celebration recipes will shine through, giving you a full house of special occasion choices. There are also recipes for some exceptionally delicious puddings. As you'd expect with The Full Diet, these desserts do not contain artificial sweeteners, which is unusual for a low-sugar cookbook. I am really proud that these recipes will be a joyful addition to your celebration table, while still remaining true to your Programme principles.

There are some suggested Celebration menus on pages 256–7, but really it's up to you to decide what works for you and your festivities, drawing in dishes from other sections of the book too if that feels right for you. As with all the recipes in the book, adjust the quantities depending on how many people you are serving.

A central mission of The Full Diet is to reconnect you with the joy of togetherness and taking part. I hope you love these Celebration recipes every bit as much as my patients and I do. In time, like us, you are likely to build up some 'classics' so that when it's you hosting, everyone is hoping for your twice-baked cheese soufflé (page 182) or key lime pie (page 192).

I have taken groups through The Full Diet at every time of year, so I've become attuned to particular seasonal considerations. The first thing we do as a celebration draws near is to re-think what we mean by a 'treat'. My patients become so used to feeling healthy and energetic that drinking too much at Christmas or eating lots of chocolate at Easter no longer feels like a 'treat'. Instead we can embrace what these occasions and celebrations are really about – family, friends and connection, which are the real treats that make you feel good and fill you up emotionally.

You can also continue to eat really well at social events and special times of year by only eating the good stuff, which means enjoying the delicious lamb kleftiko (page 170) on Easter Sunday, followed by the velvety richness of chocolate mousse (page 195) while avoiding ultra-processed sugary chocolate eggs. I am often asked for suggestions in place of birthday cake. Any of the puddings in this section will work well, and if you are a summer baby, the celebration watermelon layer cake (page 188) is a stunning table centrepiece as well as a fresh taste sensation.

As you would expect, Christmas in our December groups is always a talking point, and some of my patients ask how they can enjoy the day while continuing towards their Programme goals. My advice is always: don't worry, Christmas lunch is just a big roast. When we reconvene in January, they confirm this was correct!

What I mean by this is that the main event for many of us is the turkey. Make a flavoured herby butter and put it under the skin of the bird, season with salt and pepper, baste while cooking to keep moist, and use the pan juices to make gravy. Fill the turkey cavity with the stuffing on page 156 and bake the remaining stuffing separately in a roasting tin. If you'd prefer a vegetarian option, you can substitute the sausagemeat with chestnuts and mushrooms, chopped up small and then browned up before being added. This stuffing is also a perfect side. If you'd prefer a non-meat-based Christmas lunch, the roast butternut squash (page 177) is a rich and warming alternative. Serve your Christmas lunch with any veggie sides in the book, and customize as needed. For example, celeriac chips (page 220) cut into larger chunks make a great alternative to roast potatoes. Any sides such as pigs in blankets, roast Brussels sprouts (page 221) or cauliflower cheese wedges (page 215) finish things off beautifully. Your fullness hormone signal will certainly be strong when you finish. Then, later on, when your ghrelin hunger signal begins to return, a cheeseboard with crunchy crudités is a perfect end to the meal.

But why have all this know-how up your sleeve? Surely special events are just that, special and one-off, so why not go off-piste and then get back on the Programme tomorrow? The issue with this approach is that not only could you backtrack with stalled weight loss or even re-gain, but cravings, especially for sweet things, can quickly return. You might be wondering, would this really happen if I occasionally go to an event and eat off-Programme? The answer here is that it depends what you mean by 'occasionally'.

Working with my patients has shown me that people lead full, busy, active lives with work, family, friends and travel. Because of this, rather than 'occasionally', in fact they have many opportunities in an average week when they could choose to make an exception. These events could be any of the following: a work party, a colleague's leaving drinks, a conference, a family lunch, a weekend away, an anniversary, a birthday, a wedding, going to a special restaurant, a holiday, Valentine's, Easter, Hallowe'en, Bonfire Night, Christmas and New Year, as well as celebrations important to you and your family like Diwali, Hanukah and Eid.

By running my patient groups throughout the year, I have seen that for many people, exceptional events aren't in fact exceptional at all. When our patient groups reframe these occasions, from off-Programme events into an opportunity to enjoy all the incredible Full Diet food that is propelling them toward their weight loss and wellbeing goals, these events become all the more special.

Classic roast chicken with sausage and sage stuffing

Serves 4–6

Takes approx. 1 hour 45 minutes (depending on the weight of the chicken)

Hands-on: 30 minutes
Hands-off: 1 hour 15 minutes

A timeless favourite, this roast chicken speaks of home and togetherness. The stuffing is brilliantly versatile and can be used as a side for any dish you choose, and it's delicious with turkey for Christmas done The Full Diet way.

See picture on page 158.

For the chicken

1 large chicken (approx. 1.8kg)

olive oil, for drizzling

salt and black pepper

For the stuffing

100g toasted pine nuts

20g butter

1 tablespoon olive oil

2 red onions, thinly sliced

800g pork sausagemeat

1 large Bramley apple, peeled, core removed and cut into cubes

2 tablespoons sage leaves, chopped

1 tablespoon chopped parsley or tarragon

2 cloves of garlic, peeled and finely grated

½ teaspoon ground or freshly grated nutmeg

1 unwaxed lemon, zest only

olive oil

salt and black pepper

Take the chicken out the fridge 1 hour before you are going to cook it. Take it out of any plastic packaging, cover with kitchen paper and let it come up to room temperature.

Preheat the oven to 210°C/190°C fan/gas 6 and line a roasting tin with baking paper.

To make the stuffing, first toast the pine nuts by placing them in a frying pan or skillet over a medium heat for 2–3 minutes, shaking the pan frequently until the pine nuts just start to brown. Make sure to keep a close eye on them as they can burn easily. Remove from the heat.

Heat the butter and olive oil in a large frying pan and add the sliced red onions. Cook with a pinch of salt on a low heat until softened and starting to turn golden – this will take around 15–20 minutes. Add the pine nuts and cook for another 10 minutes. Allow to cool slightly.

Place the sausagemeat in a bowl with the grated apple, sage, parsley, garlic, nutmeg, lemon zest and some black pepper. Add the onions and pine nuts and use your hands to mix it all together.

Place roughly a third of the stuffing in the cavity of the bird and the rest in a shallow roasting dish greased with a little butter. Wash your hands thoroughly after handling the raw sausagemeat.

Put the chicken into the lined roasting tin, drizzle over a little olive oil and season generously with salt and pepper.

Put the roasting tin into the oven. The cooking time of the chicken will depend on the weight, so check the instructions on the label.

An hour before the chicken is due to come out, place the dish of stuffing in the oven on the shelf underneath and roast for an hour.

Once the time is up, remove from the oven and check the chicken is cooked through (all the meat should be white and opaque and the juices should run clear) and allow to rest for 15 minutes before carving. Pour the juices from the roasting tin into a jug to pour over the chicken at the table.

Serve the chicken alongside the stuffing, the juices in the jug and vegetable sides of your choosing.

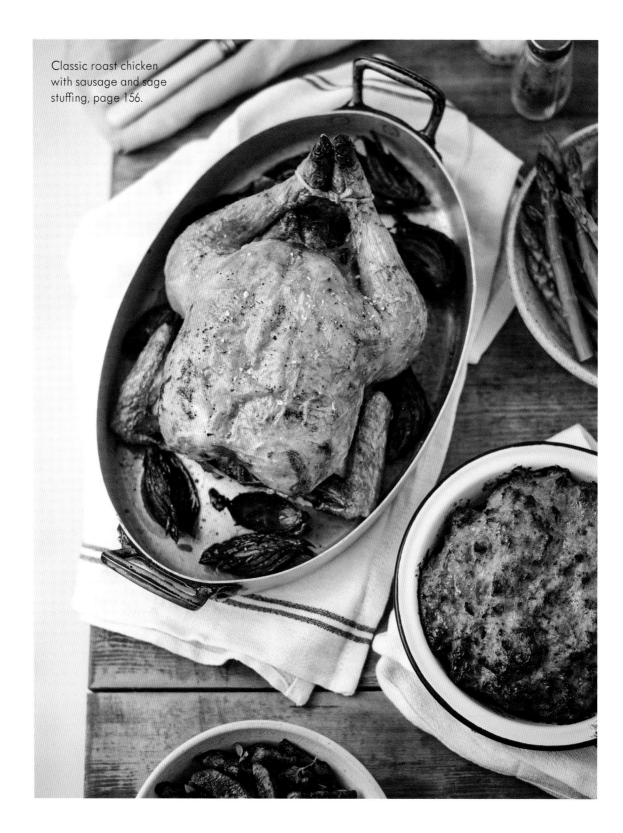

Classic roast chicken with sausage and sage stuffing, page 156.

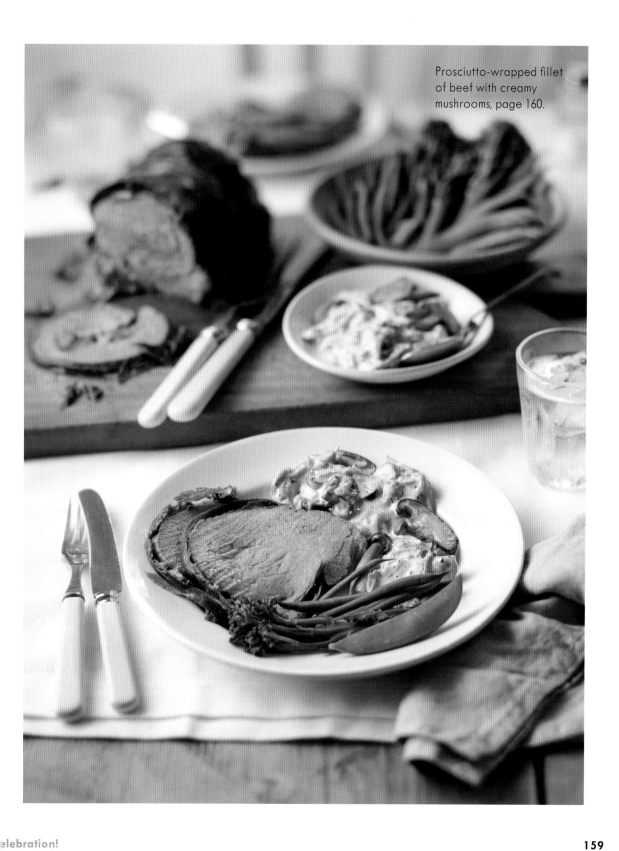

Prosciutto-wrapped fillet of beef with creamy mushrooms, page 160.

Prosciutto-wrapped fillet of beef with creamy mushrooms

Serves 6

Takes 40–70 minutes (depending how you like your beef cooked)

Hands-on: 10–15 minutes
Hands-off: 30–55 minutes

This is a special recipe for a special meal — buttery soft beef fillet with the richness of creamy mushrooms, to be enjoyed with people whose souls you want to fill up. This dish would be just as happy on the menu at a top restaurant as in *The Full Diet Cookbook*. That's the beauty of the Programme, which sees food as a pleasure, with the power to bring people together while quietly giving you all the good health you seek.

See picture on previous page.

For the fillet

1.5kg fillet of beef or topside, from the middle so it's an even width for cooking

10g butter

1 tablespoon olive oil

12 slices of prosciutto

1 teaspoon Dijon mustard

salt and black pepper

For the mushrooms

40g butter

2 tablespoons olive oil

4 banana shallots, peeled, halved and thinly sliced into half-moon shapes, layers separated

1 teaspoon chopped fresh thyme leaves

1 teaspoon chopped fresh tarragon

400g mushrooms, such as chestnut or portabellini

350ml double cream

salt and black pepper

For the horseradish

4 tablespoons fresh grated horseradish

2 tablespoons crème fraîche

2 tablespoons double cream

1–2 teaspoons lemon juice

salt

1 teaspoon chopped chives (optional)

Remove the beef from the fridge. Pat dry with kitchen paper and leave covered with kitchen paper for 2 hours before cooking, so it comes up to room temperature.

To make the horseradish, combine all the ingredients in a bowl and leave to set and infuse in the fridge for at least an hour before serving. When ready to serve, garnish with the chives (if using).

Preheat the oven to 210°C/190°C fan/gas 6.

Season the beef fillet generously with salt and pepper. Heat a large frying pan and add the butter and olive oil. Once the butter has melted and started foaming, add the beef and sear the outside by cooking for only a minute on each side, until browned. Remove from the heat and allow to cool.

On a sheet of baking paper, lay out the prosciutto slices, 2 slices wide and 6 slices deep, each overlapping with the other.

Rub the mustard over the outside of the beef, then lay the fillet on top of the prosciutto and wrap the prosciutto over the beef, with the ends of the prosciutto overlapping where they meet.

Place the beef in a roasting tin and cook in the oven for 30 minutes if you like your beef rare; for medium rare 35 minutes, medium 40 minutes and well done 50 minutes. When the cooking time is completed, remove the beef from the oven and allow to rest for 15 minutes before carving.

While the beef is resting, cook the mushrooms. Reheat the frying pan that you used for the beef on a high heat and add the butter and oil. Add the shallots and cook for a couple of minutes until they start to soften and turn golden. Add the fresh herbs and mushrooms and cook until they start to take on some colour. Add the cream, bring to the boil, then reduce the heat and just simmer for about 6–8 minutes until you are ready to serve the beef.

Carve the beef into thin slices and serve with the prosciutto, mushrooms and horseradish, and some steamed green vegetables.

Porchetta

Serves 8–10

Takes 4 hours 30 minutes, plus chilling time

Hands-on: 30 minutes
Hands-off: 4 hours

3.5kg pork loin with belly attached (will be approx. 5kg with the bones in)

3 tablespoons roughly chopped parsley

1 tablespoon thyme leaves

2 teaspoons rosemary leaves

8 cloves of garlic

salt and black pepper

To serve

apple sauce (page 235)

Hours of slow cooking infuse the herbs and garlic into this Italian classic rolled pork, while the meat quietly roasts until it is melt-in-the-mouth good. Served with salty, fatty crackling and a cauliflower cheese side, this perennially popular favourite makes a beautiful table centrepiece, ideal for special celebrations and festivities.

Ask the butcher to prepare your meat for you. The skin on the belly section needs to be removed, and the skin on the loin needs to be scored.

Lay out the meat on a large chopping board, skin side down.

Place all the other ingredients in a mini chopper or the small bowl of a food processor, and blitz to a paste. You can also use a mortar and pestle, if you don't have an electric blender. Spread the paste over the flesh, then roll up the meat from the belly side into a roulade shape and use butcher's string to tie it up at 5cm intervals to hold it in the round shape.

Rub a generous amount of salt into the skin, which really helps to crisp it up. Wash your hands thoroughly after handling raw meat. Lightly cover the pork with kitchen paper and chill in the fridge for 1–2 hours. This dries out the skin by removing the moisture and allows for the skin to become really good crunchy crackling.

Remove the porchetta from the fridge and keep it covered as it comes up to room temperature. Preheat the oven to 180°C/160°C fan/gas 4. Uncover the porchetta, place in a large roasting tray and roast in the oven for 4 hours. It will take care of itself completely, so you don't need to pay it any attention until the time is up.

When the time is up, remove from the oven and leave the porchetta to rest for 10–15 minutes before serving in slices along with the crackling. Delicious served with cauliflower cheese wedges (page 215), apple sauce (page 235) and simple steamed greens like green beans or broccoli.

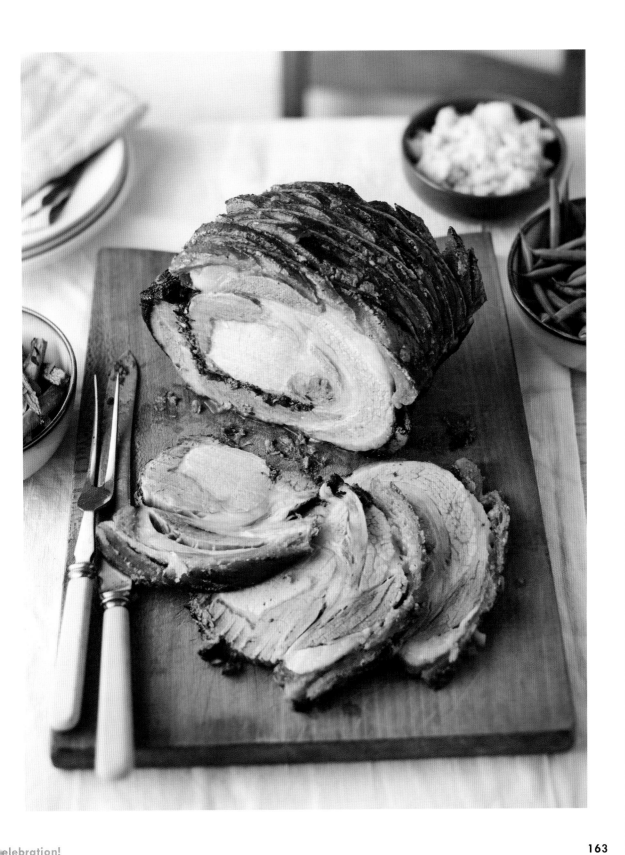

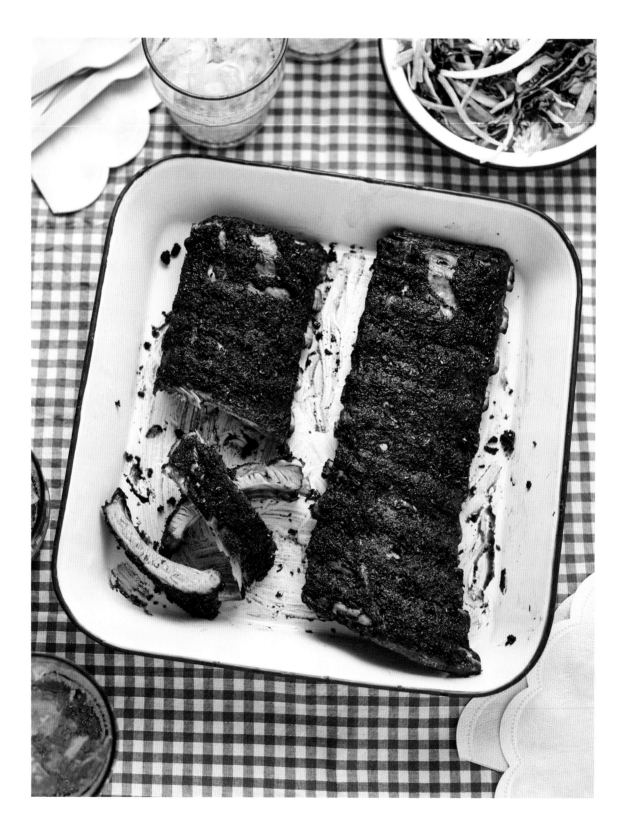

celebration

Sticky finger barbecue ribs

Serves 4

Takes 3 hours,
plus marinating time

Hands-on: 30 minutes
Hands-off: 2 hours 30 minutes

These melt-in-the-mouth ribs coated in caramelized smoky barbecue sauce are lip-smackingly good. There is no other way to eat them than with your fingers – a napkin tucked into your collar also tends to come in handy.

2 racks of baby back pork ribs (approx. 700g)

4 tablespoons homemade ketchup (page 236)

2 tablespoons barbecue rub (see below)

For the barbecue rub (makes more rub than you need, store in an airtight tub for up to 3 months)

2 tablespoons dried oregano

2 tablespoons sweet smoked paprika

1½ tablespoons garlic powder

1½ tablespoons onion powder

1 tablespoon sea salt

2 teaspoons chipotle chilli flakes

1½ teaspoons ground coriander

½ teaspoon dried thyme

½ teaspoon ground or freshly grated nutmeg

½ teaspoon black pepper

Place all the rub ingredients in a Tupperware-type container, replace the lid and shake to combine.

Line a large roasting tin with tin foil and place the ribs on top. Add the ketchup and barbecue rub and use your hands to rub everything all over the ribs so that they are well coated. Wash your hands thoroughly after handling the raw meat. Cover the tin with a second piece of tin foil and chill in the fridge for at least 2 hours, for the rub flavours to infuse into the meat, or ideally over-night if possible.

Take the roasting tin out of the fridge about an hour before cooking and let the ribs come up to room temperature.

Preheat the oven to 170°C/150°C fan/gas 3.

Place in the oven for 2½ hours. Once the time is up, remove from the oven and uncover.

Heat your grill to its maximum setting (or finish on the barbecue) and grill the ribs. Cook the top and bottom sides for 3–4 minutes each, until you start to get some good colour on them.

Slice and serve alongside any barbecue sides that you like, for example super crunchy rainbow slaw (page 202) or a crisp green salad.

Pulled pork lettuce wraps

Serves 4

Takes 3 hours 45 minutes, plus marinating time

Hands-on: 15 minutes
Hands-off: 3 hours 30 minutes

1.5kg pork shoulder (in one piece, skin removed and off the bone)

2 tablespoons barbecue rub (page 165)

To serve

1 large romaine or cos lettuce, base trimmed and leaves pulled apart

4 chopped gherkins

4 tomatoes, diced

100ml sour cream

100g Cheddar, grated

2 tablespoons chopped fresh coriander

pow-pow! chilli sauce (page 237) (optional)

This smoky pulled pork is a perfect alternative to a roast joint. Impossible to eat neatly, these are perfect for relaxed entertaining. Pile them high with all the extras, then relax into every last finger-licking bite.

Take a casserole dish and put in the meat. Add the rub and use your hands to cover the meat on all sides. Wash your hands thoroughly after handling raw meat.

Put the lid on the casserole dish and refrigerate for at least two hours (or ideally overnight) to let the rub flavour infuse into the pork.

Take the casserole out of the fridge and allow the meat to come up to room temperature. Preheat the oven to 170°C/150°C fan/gas 3, then, keeping the lid on the casserole dish, put in the oven and cook for 3½ hours.

Remove from the oven and take the meat out of the pan. Remove any excess fat from the pan by absorbing it with kitchen paper or pouring it off. Keep any juices.

Shred the meat with two forks and return it to the pan to keep warm.

Lay out the lettuce leaves and spoon the pulled pork on top. Serve the toppings — gherkins, tomatoes, sour cream and Cheddar, fresh coriander and pow-pow! chilli sauce (if using) — in bowls for people to pile into their wraps. Serve with a side of broccoli or green beans or any other veg of your choosing.

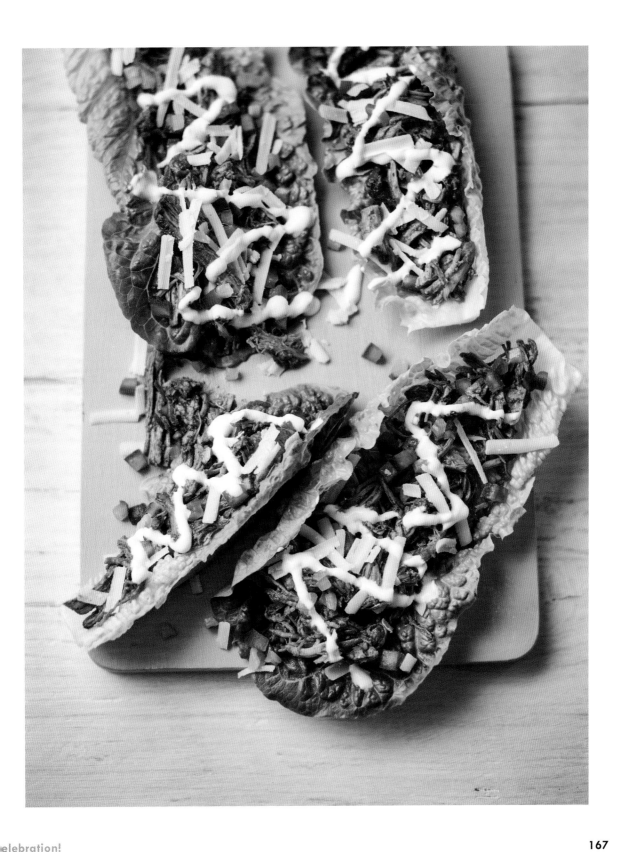

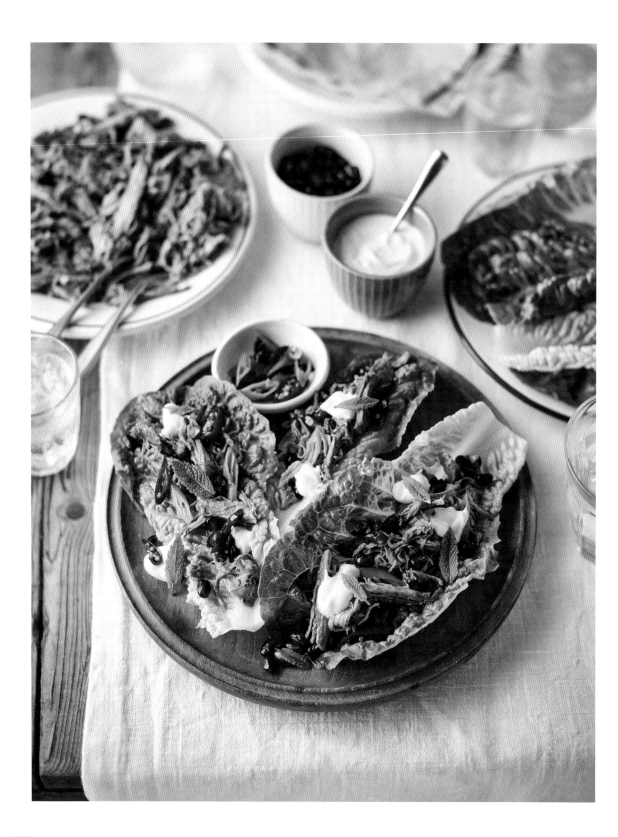

Shredded lamb lettuce wraps

Serves 6

Takes 3–3½ hours

Hands-on: 30 minutes
Hands-off: 3 hours

Slow cooking transforms a lamb shoulder into a feast of melting, fall-off-the-bone goodness. This makes a delicious and surprising alternative to a Sunday roast and is also perfect for a spring celebration – from Easter to Eid, Mother's Day to Passover, whatever you are celebrating, this dish is a triumph of good eating and togetherness.

For the lamb

4 sprigs of rosemary

1 lamb shoulder
  (approx. 2kg)

3 tablespoons olive oil

½ teaspoon garlic granules

salt and black pepper

To serve

2 romaine lettuces, base
  trimmed and bigger leaves
  pulled apart

100g full-fat Greek yoghurt

4 sprigs of mint, leaves
  picked and shredded

100g pomegranate seeds

8 pickled chillies, sliced

2 limes, juice only

black pepper

Take the lamb out of the fridge, remove any plastic packaging, cover with kitchen paper, and allow the meat to come up to room temperature.

Preheat the oven to 170°C/150°C fan/gas 3 and line a roasting tin with baking paper.

Place the rosemary sprigs on top of the baking paper, then lay the lamb shoulder on top of the rosemary sprigs. Drizzle the lamb with the olive oil, then sprinkle over the garlic granules and season with salt and black pepper. Put the tin into the oven and roast slowly for 3 hours.

After 3 hours is up, remove the roasting tin from the oven and use a fork to try and shred some of the meat. If it pulls apart easily (you're looking for the meat under the skin) it's done, but if there's still some resistance, return it to the oven for another 15 minutes and check again.

Once you are happy the meat is done, remove from the oven and allow to cool for 15 minutes, then shred the meat using two forks.

Lay out all the lettuce leaves (allow about 2–3 per person) and layer in some of the shredded meat. Using a teaspoon, spoon over a little yoghurt, scatter over the mint leaves, pomegranate seeds and pickled chilli, and finish with a squeeze of fresh lime juice and a twist of black pepper.

Lamb kleftiko

Serves 6–8

Takes 3 hours

Hands-on: 30 minutes
Hands-off: 2 hours 30 minutes

This traditional Greek parcel of sweet lamb infused with fresh oregano and pungent garlic and slow-cooked to soft, melting perfection is ideal for a springtime feast such as Easter, Passover or Mother's Day. Serve on a bed of the roasted veg and drizzle over the caramelized pan juices for a celebratory meal that memories are made of.

1 leg of lamb on the bone (approx. 2–2.5kg)

3 mixed peppers (red and yellow), deseeded and cut into wedges

2 red onions, peeled and cut into wedges

6 tomatoes, halved

8 cloves of garlic, peeled and sliced

3 tablespoons extra virgin olive oil

10 sprigs of fresh oregano

200g feta cheese

salt and black pepper

To serve

3 tablespoons chopped fresh mint

lemon wedges

extra virgin olive oil

Take the lamb out of the fridge, remove any plastic packaging, cover with kitchen paper, and allow the meat to come up to room temperature.

Preheat the oven to 180°C/160°C fan/gas 4. Take two pieces of non-stick baking paper approx. 90cm each, and place them over a large roasting tin in the shape of a cross.

Place the lamb leg in the roasting tin on top of the baking paper. Scatter the peppers, onions, tomatoes and garlic around the lamb, then drizzle the oil over everything and tuck the herbs in and around. Season all over with salt and pepper, then wrap the lamb in the paper, tucking it around and enveloping the lamb inside.

Put the roasting tin into the oven for 2 hours.

Remove the tray from the oven, open up the parcel and crumble over the feta. Turn the heat up to 220°C/200°C fan/gas 7 and, keeping the lamb uncovered, return the tin to the oven for another 30 minutes, to crisp up the skin, bake the feta and char the veg a little.

Remove from the oven and leave to rest for 15 minutes before carving.

Garnish with some fresh mint and serve the lamb alongside the roasted vegetables — some green beans or spring greens would also be delicious with this.

Serve with lemon wedges to squeeze over the lamb and some extra virgin olive oil on the table in case your guests would like an extra drizzle.

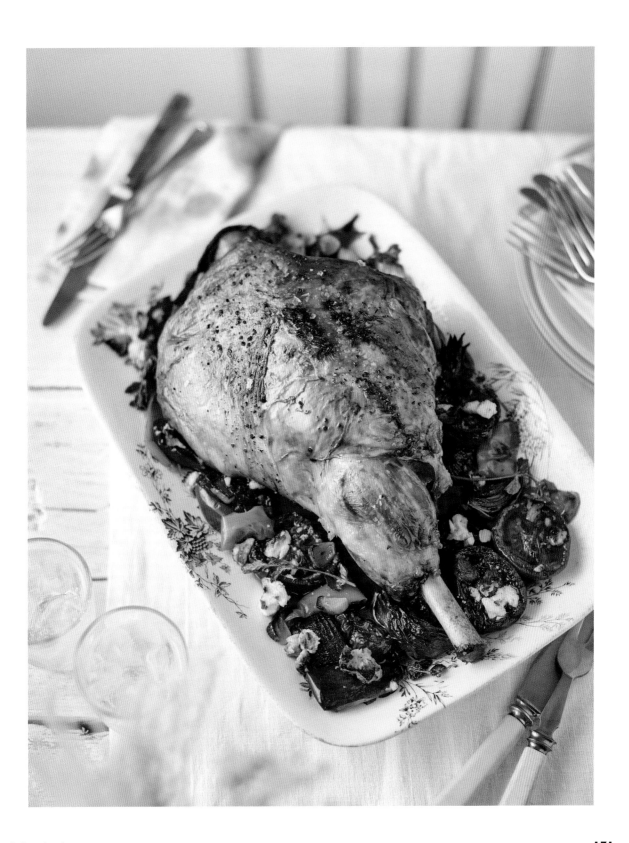

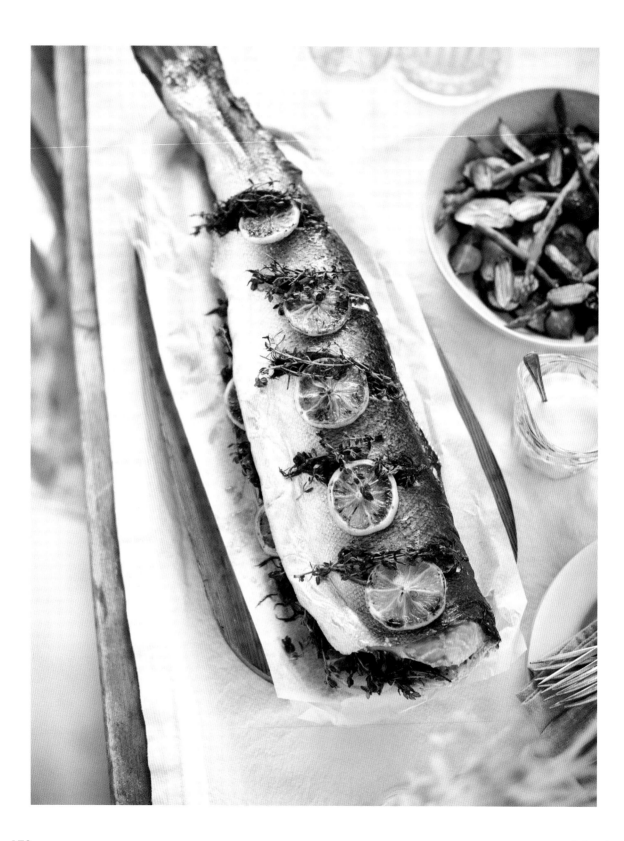

Whole lemon and herb-stuffed roast salmon with hollandaise

Serves 10–12

Takes 55 minutes

Hands-on: 10 minutes
Hands-off: 40–45 minutes

A whole roasted salmon stuffed with lemon, fresh herbs and garlic on a bed of vegetable abundance and topped with rich warm, buttery hollandaise – displayed as the centrepiece at a table of gathered loved ones, this dish is a timeless celebration wow moment.

1 whole salmon (approx. 2.5kg), scaled and gutted

1 lemon, thinly sliced

1 packet of thyme (approx. 20g)

1 packet of dill (approx. 20g)

6 cloves of garlic, peeled and crushed

1 bunch of asparagus, woody ends snapped off

1 courgette, cut into 1 cm slices

200g radishes, halved

3 tablespoons olive oil

salt and black pepper

To serve

lemon wedges

green salad leaves

hollandaise sauce (page 44), multiply these quantities by six

Preheat the oven to 240°C/220°C fan/gas 9 and line a large baking sheet with non-stick baking paper.

Squeeze the salmon into the tin – you may have to curve the head and tail around slightly, or let them protrude over the edge of the tray a little (or you could remove them if you want to).

Cut five slashes in each side of the salmon and add a slice of lemon and some thyme and dill to each one. Put the rest of the lemon and herbs and the garlic into the cavity.

Place the asparagus, courgette and radishes around the fish, then drizzle everything with the olive oil and season with salt and pepper.

Place in the very hot oven for 20 minutes, then reduce the heat to 190°C/170°C fan/gas 5 and cook for another 20–25 minutes, until the flesh is just cooked. It will be pale pink and opaque all the way through.

Carefully remove from the roasting tin, ensuring the fish remains whole, and arrange on a serving platter alongside fresh lemon wedges, the vegetables from the roasting tin and some green salad leaves.

Serve with hollandaise on the side.

Chilli and ginger whole roast sea bass

Serves 2

Takes 25 minutes

1 sea bass, gutted (for each additional pair of guests, add a fish)

1 tablespoon sesame oil

For the dressing

2 red Thai chillies, sliced

4 spring onions, very thinly sliced

2cm piece of ginger, peeled and finely grated

2 tablespoons soy sauce (check ingredients – ideally should be water, soybeans and salt only)

1 tablespoon sesame oil

1 lime, juice only

1 tablespoon sesame seeds

This aromatic roasted sea bass balances a perfect harmony of sweet ginger, salty soy sauce, chilli heat and sesame seed crunch. It is the ideal synergy of being gorgeously easy, yet always special at a celebratory table.

Preheat the oven to 220°C/200°C fan/gas 7 and line a roasting tin with non-stick baking paper.

Lay the fish in the tin and make a few slashes into the flesh on both sides. Drizzle over the sesame oil and rub it all over the fish. Roast in the oven for 15–20 minutes, until the fish is cooked through.

While the fish is roasting, mix all the ingredients for the dressing and keep to one side.

Once the fish is done, pour over the dressing and allow it to absorb all the flavours for 10 minutes before serving.

This is delicious served with crisp, crunchy greens like sugar snap peas or mangetout, or serve with cauliflower rice (page 216).

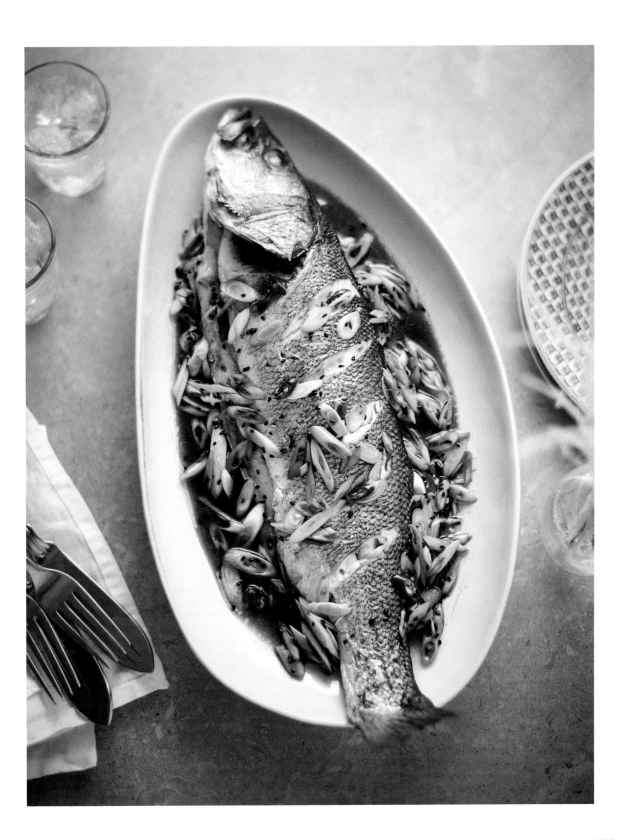

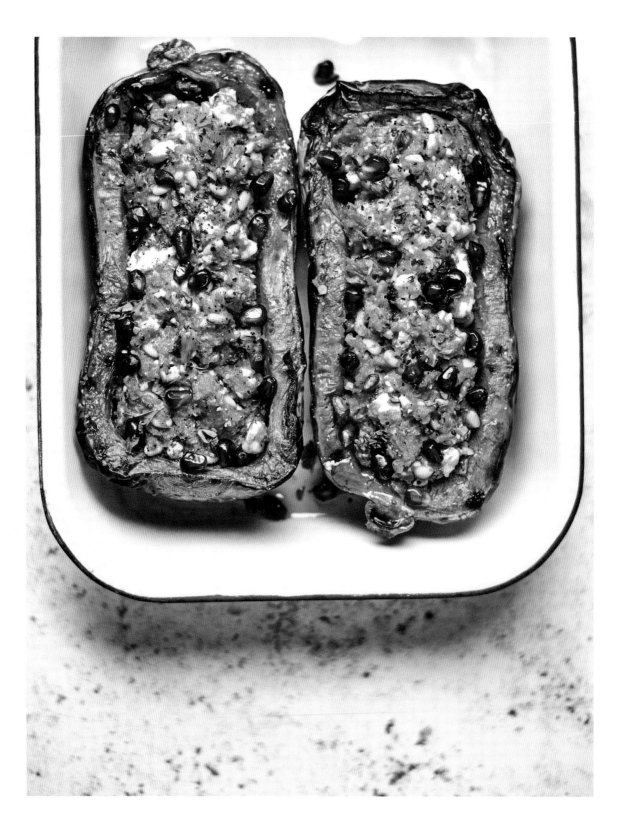

Roast butternut squash

**Serves 4 as a side
or 2 as a main**

Takes 1 hour 25 minutes

Hands-on: 15 minutes
Hands-off: 1 hour 10 minutes

Squash is a slightly starchier option, so it will raise the blood sugar more than other vegetables. That said, enjoying its vibrant colour and nutty flavour now and again will work just fine. This is a dish of contrasts — the soft sticky squash brought alive by the crunch of the nuts, the salty feta all beautifully balanced by the sweet pomegranate seeds. Enjoy as a main or a side, or carry as a portable option or to share as part of a picnic spread.

1 butternut squash, cut in half lengthways, seeds removed

1 tablespoon olive oil

100g feta, crumbled

20g pine nuts, toasted

20g walnuts, roughly chopped

1 tablespoon chopped parsley

1 tablespoon extra virgin olive oil

30g pomegranate seeds

salt and black pepper

To serve

rocket leaves or butter lettuce

Preheat the oven to 200°C/180°C fan/gas 6 and line a roasting tin with baking paper.

Lay the two halves of the butternut squash in the tin and brush the olive oil over the cut side. Season with a little salt and pepper and roast for 1 hour.

While the squash is roasting, put the feta, pine nuts, walnuts and parsley into a mixing bowl and toss with the extra virgin olive oil.

The squash should be tender all the way through, or very close to it, after an hour in the oven. If you need to, return it to the oven for another 10 minutes and check again.

Once the squash is tender, remove it from the oven. Use a spoon to scoop out some of the flesh (you want to leave about a centimetre of thickness behind) and add it to the mixing bowl with the feta and nuts. Stir to combine.

Fill the hollows of the butternut squash with the feta mix and pile it up. Return to the oven for 10 minutes, then remove, place on a serving plate and scatter over the pomegranate seeds.

This is delicious served with some rocket or butter lettuce or any other leaves with a bit of acidity which will cut through the gorgeous richness of the roasted squash.

Chilli con butternut

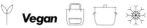 **Vegan**

Serves 8–10

Takes 50 minutes

Hands-on: 20 minutes
Hands-off: 30 minutes

This chilli, rich with coffee and chocolate has a sensational depth of flavour, perfect when cooking for a crowd or for a special occasion like Hallowe'en or Bonfire Night. Please don't be put off by the long list of ingredients. Like me, you might find the chopping quietly meditative, and once done, the rest is mainly a case of adding and stirring. I like to serve this in a huge decorative bowl, with the sour cream, avocado and grated cheese in separate dishes for everyone to help themselves.

See picture on page 180.

1 large butternut squash, peeled, seeds removed, cut into 2cm chunks

4 tablespoons olive oil

1 teaspoon ground cinnamon

400g tin of mixed beans, drained and rinsed

400g tin of black beans, drained and rinsed

1 onion, diced

1 large red pepper, 1 large yellow pepper and 1 large green pepper, all deseeded and cut into chunks

1 tablespoon oregano

1 tablespoon sweet smoked paprika

1 teaspoon chilli flakes (or to taste)

1 teaspoon ground cumin

5 cloves of garlic, peeled and grated

100g tomato purée

250g ready-cooked lentils (tinned or packet)

640ml passata

400g tin of chopped tomatoes

100ml espresso

3 squares of 90% dark chocolate

extra virgin olive oil

3 tablespoons chopped coriander

salt and black pepper

To serve

300ml sour cream

3 avocados, sliced

300g Cheddar, grated

Preheat the oven to 200°C/180°C fan/gas 6 and line a roasting tin with baking paper.

Put the butternut squash into the roasting tin and drizzle over half the olive oil, the cinnamon and some salt and pepper. Toss to coat. Roast for 25–30 minutes, until tender and golden at the edges.

While the squash is roasting, tip the mixed beans and the black beans into a sieve or colander set over the sink and rinse for about 30 seconds under the cold tap, until the water draining off runs clear.

Heat the remaining oil in a large casserole pot on a medium heat and add the onion and peppers. Cook for 15 minutes, until softening, then add the spices, garlic and tomato purée.

Add the beans, lentils, passata and chopped tomatoes, along with the espresso and chocolate. Stir to combine, then bring to a simmer. Stir occasionally while you are waiting for the butternut squash.

Once the squash is cooked, tip it into the pot of chilli, and gently stir to combine. Try not to break up the squash too much.

Before serving, drizzle over some extra virgin olive oil and garnish with fresh coriander.

Serve with bowls of sour cream, avocado and Cheddar for your guests to add their own toppings.

This chilli goes really well with cauliflower rice, (page 216) green beans or any other green vegetable you like.

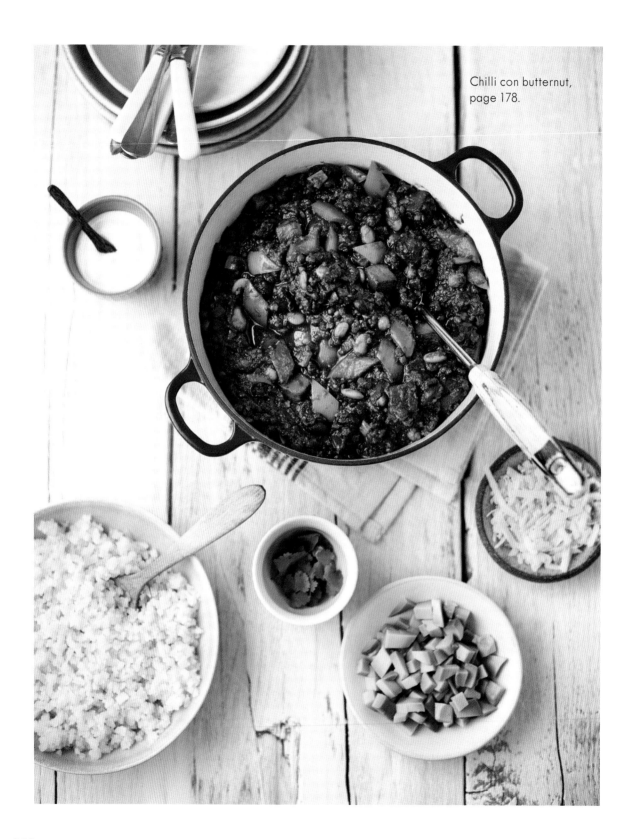

Chilli con butternut,
page 178.

celebration

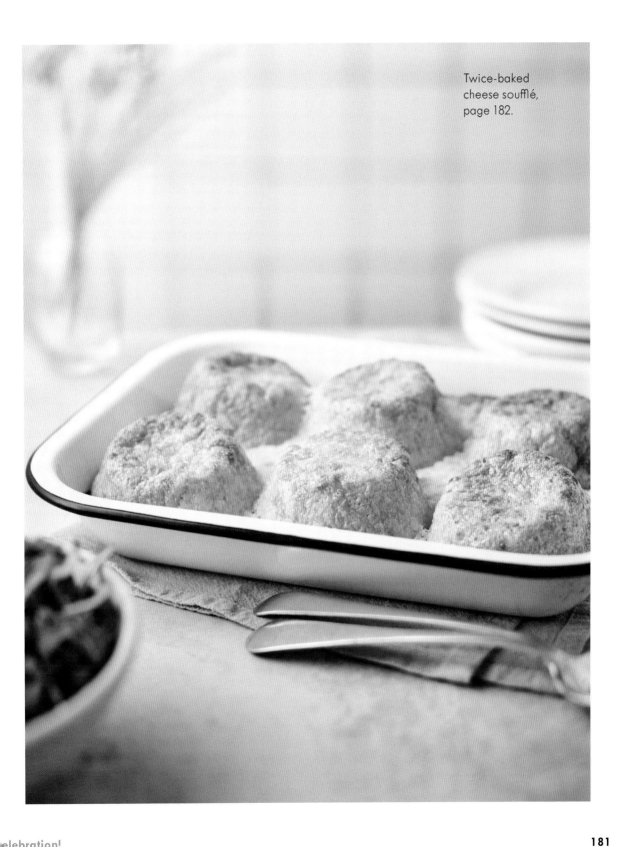

Twice-baked
cheese soufflé,
page 182.

Twice-baked cheese soufflé

(if vegetarian Parmesan used)

Serves 6

Takes 40 minutes

My best friend's mother used to insist on total silence when a soufflé was baking, sure that too much noise would lead to a collapse. If you have similar worries that soufflés are difficult (and sensitive) – rest assured, this one is not. The cheese mix is easy to whiz up, and the twice-baking gives a depth of flavour that belies the ease of production. Serve with peppery rocket, which contrasts beautifully with the rich, creamy soufflés.

See picture on previous page.

For the ramekins

butter

3 tablespoons grated Parmesan

For the soufflés

50g butter

2 teaspoons arrowroot powder

120ml whole milk

120ml double cream

200g strong cheese, such as Gruyère, grated

4 eggs, separated into yolks and whites

2 tablespoons finely chopped soft herbs, such as parsley, chives, tarragon or basil

salt and black pepper

To finish

250ml double cream

50g Parmesan, grated

To serve

rocket leaves

Preheat the oven to 180°C/160°C fan/gas 4. Grease 6 ramekins with butter and sprinkle the Parmesan round the inside, to stick to the butter.

Place a large roasting tin on your worktop and sit the ramekins in it. Carefully fill the tin with water until it is halfway up the sides of the ramekins. Remove the ramekins and place the tin in the oven.

Heat the butter in a saucepan over a medium heat, then add the arrowroot powder and stir together into a paste. Add the milk slowly, whisking as you go, followed by the cream. Keep cooking until you have a thick sauce. Remove from the heat.

Add the grated cheese and stir until it has melted into the sauce. Add the egg yolks and again, whisk gently to combine.

Beat the egg whites to stiff peaks (which means they stand up on their own). Use a large metal spoon to fold the egg whites into the cheese mix, along with some salt and pepper and the herbs of your choice.

Divide the soufflé mixture between the 6 ramekins – the mix should come up to the top. Level off with a spatula, then place the ramekins in the water-filled roasting tin and cook in the oven for around 18–20 minutes, until they are golden brown and risen.

Remove the roasting tin from the oven (be careful as the water inside is very hot). Use oven gloves to remove the ramekins from the roasting tin, then tip the soufflés out of the ramekins into a lightly greased ovenproof dish about 20cm x 30cm (the top of each soufflé now becomes the base). Pour over the double cream, which will also drip down the sides forming a sea of cream in which the soufflés will be sitting. Sprinkle over the Parmesan and bake again for around 10 minutes, until everything is golden and bubbling.

Serve immediately, alongside crisp rocket leaves

Whole roast queen cauliflower

**Serves 4 as a main
or 6 as a side**

Takes 1 hour 30 minutes

Hands-on: 10 minutes
Hands-off: 1 hour 20 minutes

When it comes to a plant-based wow dish, this roast cauliflower is queen of the table. Dressed in a sesame, chilli marinade with a lemon zing, and crowned with fresh herbs and jewelled pomegranate seeds, this slow-roasted cauliflower adds a majestic touch to any special occasion.

For the cauliflower

1 cauliflower, base
   trimmed to make it
   flat and big leaves
   removed

3 tablespoons olive
   oil

1 tablespoon dried
   oregano

1 tablespoon sumac

1 teaspoon garlic
   granules

½ teaspoon sea salt

½ teaspoon black
   pepper

For the dressing

150g full-fat Greek
   yoghurt

1 tablespoon tahini

1 lemon, juice only
   (to taste)

1 teaspoon chilli
   flakes (if you like
   it milder, use
   ½ teaspoon or
   alternatively
   1 teaspoon Aleppo
   chilli flakes)

salt and black
   pepper

To serve

fresh soft herbs, such
   as parsley, or
   coriander

pomegranate seeds

Preheat the oven to 200°C/180°C fan/gas 6. Place a piece of baking paper in the base of a casserole dish.

Place the cauliflower on a chopping board. Mix all the other cauliflower ingredients together in a bowl, then pour them over the cauliflower. Use your hands to rub the mix all over and into all the creases.

Put the cauliflower into the casserole, cover with the lid and bake for 1 hour. Remove the lid and continue cooking for another 20–30 minutes, until the cauliflower is tender through its core when pierced with a sharp knife.

While the cauliflower is cooking, whisk together all the ingredients for the dressing.

Transfer the cauliflower to a chopping board and cut into 4–6 wedges. Drizzle some dressing over each wedge, then scatter over the fresh herbs and pomegranate seeds. Serve the extra dressing in a jug on the table for guests who want that little bit more.

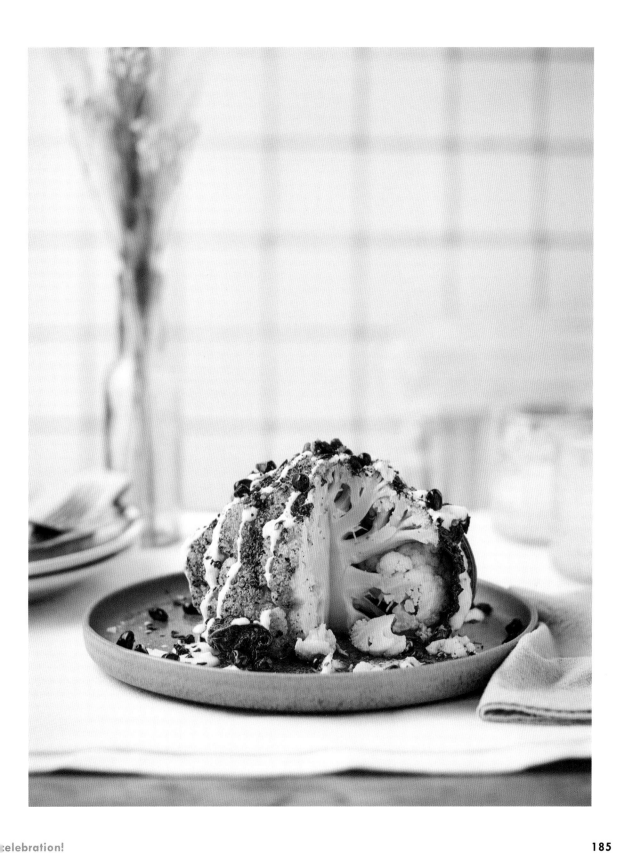

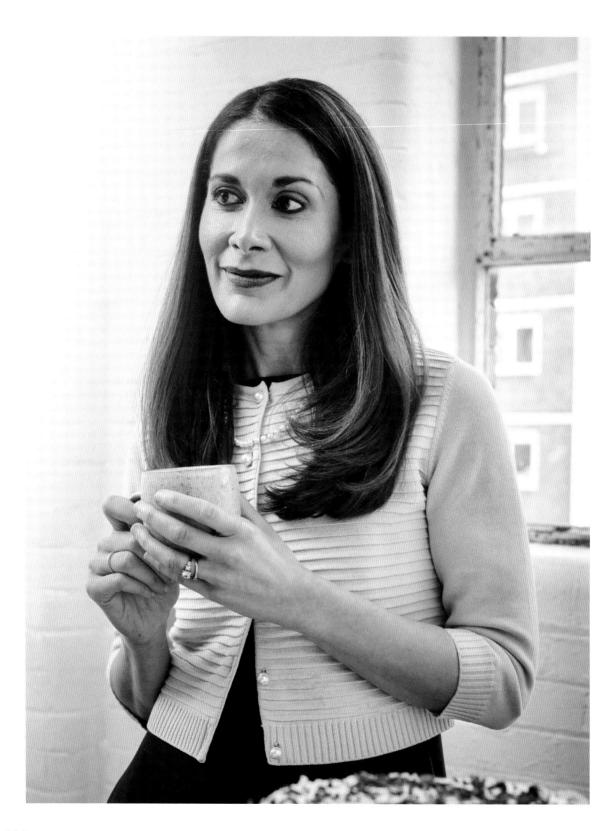

Cinnamon nut crunch apple crumble

Serves 6–8

Takes 1 hour

Hands-on: 10 minutes
Hands-off: 50 minutes

Perfect for a Hallowe'en or Bonfire Night pudding, or for eating after Sunday lunch, this warming apple crumble, spiced with sweet, fragrant cinnamon, is always a crowd-pleaser. Delicious served piping hot from the oven, cooled by a generous helping of thick, cold double cream or tangy Greek yoghurt.

For the fruit

4 Bramley apples, peeled and cut into chunks

300g blackberries

½ teaspoon ground cinnamon

For the nut crunch topping

200g ground almonds

100g pecans, chopped

50g walnuts, chopped

50g mixed seeds

3 teaspoons ground cinnamon

1 teaspoon ground ginger

80g unsalted butter (at room temperature)

To serve

full-fat Greek yoghurt or double cream

Preheat the oven to 190°C/170°C fan/gas 5.

Lightly butter a baking dish approx. 15cm x 20cm. Add the apples, blackberries and cinnamon and toss to coat, then level the fruit out in the dish.

To make the topping, put all the ingredients into a mixing bowl and use your fingers to rub the butter in. Once everything is combined, top the fruit with the nut crumble mixture.

Place the dish in the oven and cook for 30 minutes. Spin the dish around in the oven and cook for another 20 minutes, until the fruit is tender.

Serve hot, with a generous helping of yoghurt or double cream.

Celebration watermelon layer cake

Serves 12

Takes 15 minutes

1 watermelon (approx. 1kg), fridge cold

300g full-fat Greek yoghurt

800g raspberries

800g strawberries, sliced

400g blueberries

3 tablespoons small mint leaves

100g almonds, 100g pecans, 50g hazelnuts, roasted (see page 260 for instructions) and chopped

6 squares of 85% or 90% dark chocolate

This is a stunning centrepiece dessert for your table. Refreshing, beautiful to look at, full of sweetness, and a joyful splash of colour. It would be lovely as a birthday cake – just pop a candle in – it also makes the perfect pudding for a summer party.

Make the watermelon cake when you are ready to serve. You can prep the fruit and roast and chop the nuts in advance, then assemble the cake just before serving.

Cut 2cm-thick rounds from the main body of the watermelon, leaving the rind intact.

Cut each round into 6 wedges and place on a large serving board. Top each slice with yoghurt, berries, mint leaves and the chopped nuts, and finally grate the dark chocolate all over.

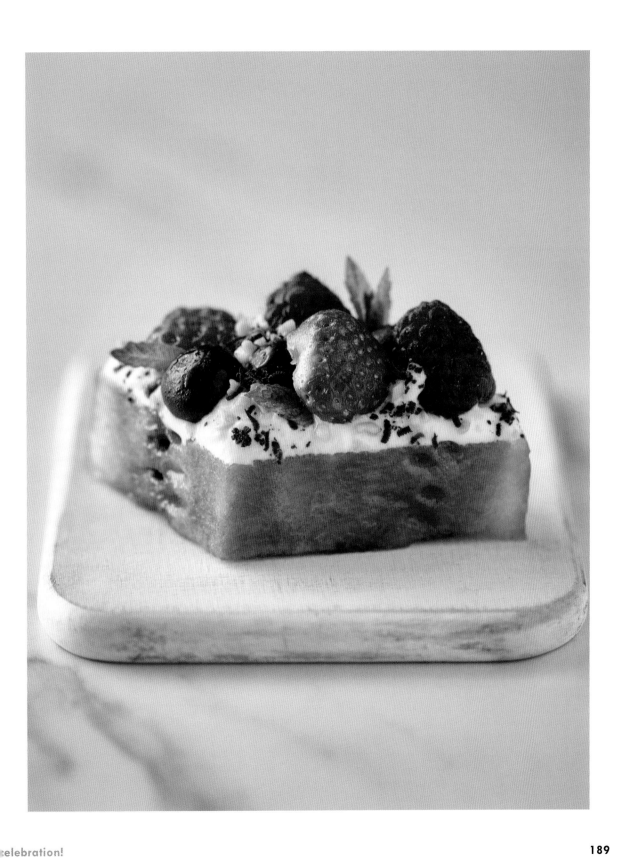

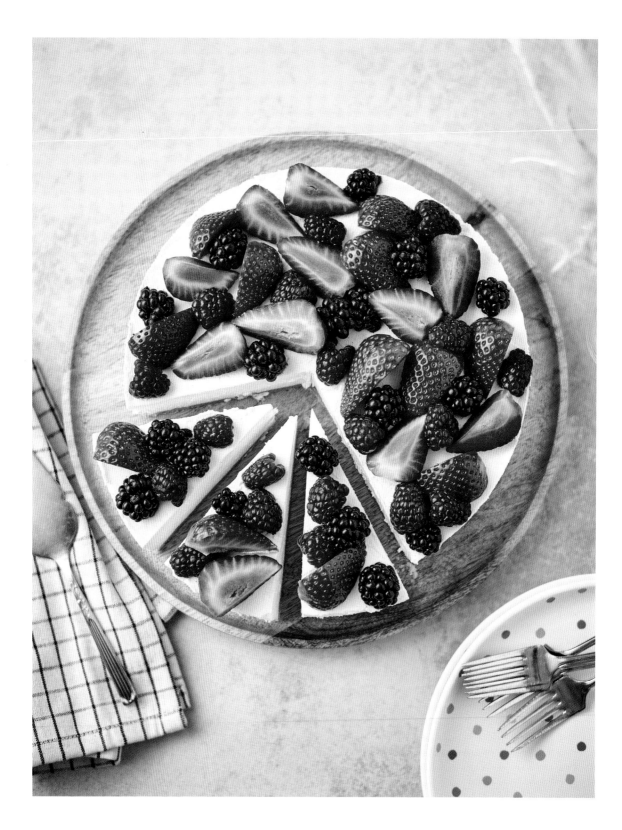

No-bake summer berry cheesecake

Serves 8–10

Takes 20 minutes,
plus chilling time

My, this looks good! Creamy, chilled cheesecake adorned with fresh berry jewels, brilliant for a summer party or served as a gorgeous birthday cake – enjoy!

For the base

150g ground almonds

50g Brazil nuts, blitzed to
a crumb

50g hazelnuts, blitzed to
a crumb

85g unsalted butter, melted

2 teaspoons ground ginger

For the filling

320g cream cheese

600ml double cream

2 unwaxed lemons, zest and
juice

½ teaspoon vanilla paste or
1 vanilla pod, cut in half
lengthways, seeds scraped

To serve

approx. 800g fresh berries,
such as strawberries,
raspberries and blueberries

Line the base and sides of a 23cm spring-release, deep-sided cake tin with baking paper.

Mix the nuts, butter and ground ginger together and tip into the base of the tin. Spread out into an even layer, press down, and chill in the freezer for 15 minutes.

While the base is chilling, place the cream cheese, double cream, lemon zest, lemon juice and vanilla pod seeds into a large mixing bowl. Use an electric hand whisk to whip until thick.

Remove the base from the freezer and spread the filling over the top, levelling it all off. Chill in the fridge to set for at least 2 hours.

Remove from the fridge and pile on the fresh mixed berries, for example, raspberries, strawberries and blueberries. Refrigerate until ready to serve.

The cheesecake can be made up to the day before.

Key lime pie

Serves 8–10

Takes 20 minutes,
plus chilling time

This zesty, creamy filled pie resting on a buttery nut crust is a perennial Full Diet favourite, ideal for parties and entertaining.

For the base

150g ground almonds

100g pecans, blitzed
to a crumb

85g unsalted butter, melted

1 tablespoon ground
cinnamon

For the filling

250g mascarpone

600ml double cream

2 unwaxed limes, zest and
juice

1 teaspoon vanilla paste or
2 vanilla pods, cut in half
lengthways, seeds scraped

To serve

4 squares of 85% or 90%
dark chocolate, for grating

lime zest

Line the base and sides of a 23cm spring-release, deep-sided cake tin with baking paper.

Mix together the nuts, butter and cinnamon, then tip into the base of the tin. Spread out into an even layer, press down, and chill in the freezer for 15 minutes.

While the base is chilling, place the mascarpone, double cream, lime zest and juice and vanilla paste in a large mixing bowl. Use an electric hand whisk to whip until thick.

Remove the base from the freezer and add the filling, spreading it out and levelling it all off. Chill in the fridge to set for at least 2 hours.

While the pie is chilling, grate the chocolate.

When ready to serve, remove from the fridge and grate over a little more lime zest, then sprinkle over the grated chocolate.

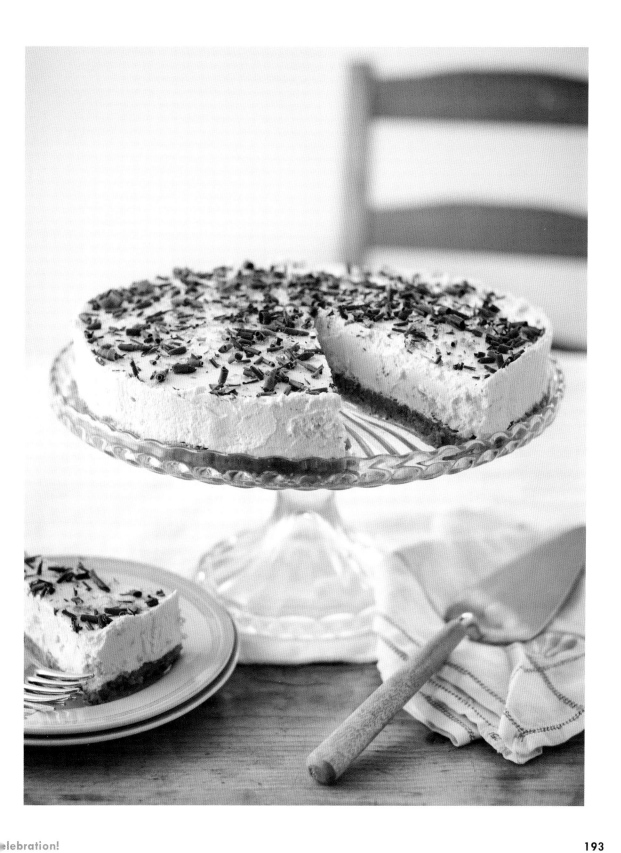

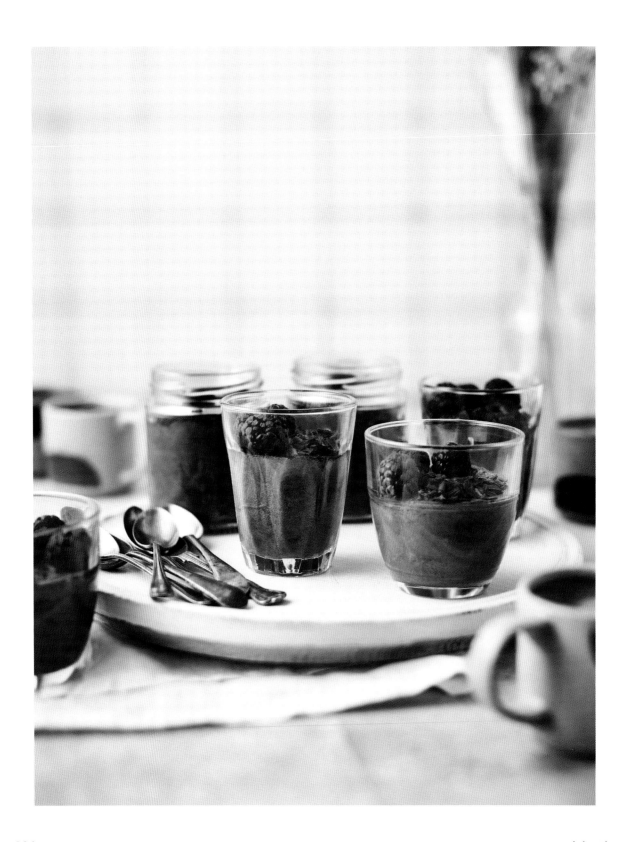

Chocolate mousse

Serves 6

Takes 10 minutes,
plus chilling time

A two-ingredient marriage made in heaven, rich dark chocolate and thick double cream, that simple, that good. Delicious served with fresh raspberries, which are perfectly refreshing eaten with the velvety, creamy mousse.

100g dark chocolate (85% or 90% cocoa solids), chopped

350ml double cream

To serve

40g dark chocolate (85% or 90% cocoa solids), grated

400g fresh raspberries

sprigs of fresh mint (optional)

Set up a bain-marie: fill a saucepan with a few centimetres of water, and place on a low heat so that the water is very gently simmering. Place a large mixing bowl on top of the saucepan and add the chocolate and 100ml of the cream to the bowl.

Stir occasionally while the chocolate melts into the cream – don't let the bowl get too hot or the mix can split – then remove from the heat and gently stir to combine.

Put the rest of the cream into another bowl and whisk, using an electric hand whisk, until it thickens, though you want it to still have some softness.

Take a large metal spoon and add a spoonful of the whipped cream to the chocolate mix. Gently fold it in, try to preserve as much of the air and volume of the whipped cream as possible. Repeat spoon by spoon until all the whipped cream is incorporated.

Divide between six glass tumblers and chill in the fridge until needed. The chocolate mouse can be made up to the day before.

When you are ready to serve, remove from the fridge, sprinkle with the grated chocolate and top with fresh raspberries and a sprig of fresh mint (if using).

sides

These delicious sides will work time and again as the perfect accompaniment to your Full Diet cooking. Of course, you might decide that one or more of these dishes deserves a starring role, in which case you can make it the main event by increasing the quantity or by adding something that will dial up even more gut-to-brain fullness, like some pulses, beans, eggs, nuts or cheese – depending on what fits best with the recipe. You can also add an extra flavour boost where you feel it will work, like a generous handful of Parmesan to melt into your broccoli mash (page 218) or a few fiery fresh red chillies to your super crunchy rainbow slaw (page 202).

These recipes are a great demonstration of how, when we broaden our horizons away from potatoes, rice, pasta and bread accompaniments, not only do we end up with controlled blood sugar, low insulin levels and fat-burning, but we also eat in a fresh, colourful and delicious way, full of flavour and variety.

Green salad

 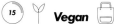 **Vegan**

Serves 2 as a side

Takes 10 minutes

This fresh, vibrant green salad is a classic accompaniment to almost any dish. Change around your choice of fresh herbs depending on what you are serving the salad with and what you have in. You can also use this recipe as a basis to make any salad you like – adding cheese, toasted nuts and seeds, boiled eggs, tuna mayo, olives, sun-dried tomatoes . . . or anything else from your delicious Full Diet kitchen.

1 cos lettuce, shredded

a large handful of rocket or watercress

a large handful of spinach leaves

¼ cucumber, cut into chunks

2 spring onions, sliced on the diagonal (optional)

1 tablespoon fresh herb leaves, such as basil, coriander, chives, parsley, tarragon, or a combination

For the dressing

2 tablespoons extra virgin olive oil

1 tablespoon white wine vinegar

1 teaspoon Dijon mustard

1 small clove of garlic, peeled and grated

salt and black pepper

To make the salad, simply toss together all the greens in a large serving bowl.

Place the ingredients for the dressing in a small bowl or clean jam jar, and whisk or shake together.

Add the dressing just before eating, to prevent the leaves going soggy.

side

G3 salad

Serves 4 as a side

Takes 10 minutes

150g green beans

150g sugar snaps

150g mangetout

1 tablespoon garlic oil

100g feta, crumbled

60g walnuts, roughly chopped

1 tablespoon nigella seeds or toasted sesame seeds

black pepper

You've heard of the G7 . . . well, the Green 3, or G3 – green beans, sugar snaps and mangetout – are even more of a powerhouse. Lots of green veg goodness offset by the rich nuttiness of the garlic oil, the tangy saltiness of the feta and the crunch of the nuts and seeds – this G3 salad means business.

Place all the green veg in a steamer basket over a pan of boiling water. Steam for 4 minutes until just tender – you want them to still have a bit of crunch but also to have a bit of give if you pierce them with a sharp knife.

Remove from the heat, drain and transfer the veg to a large serving dish. Add all the remaining ingredients and gently toss everything together. Season with freshly ground black pepper.

G3 salad is delicious eaten either hot as a side to a main meal, or cold as a great addition to a lunchbox or picnic.

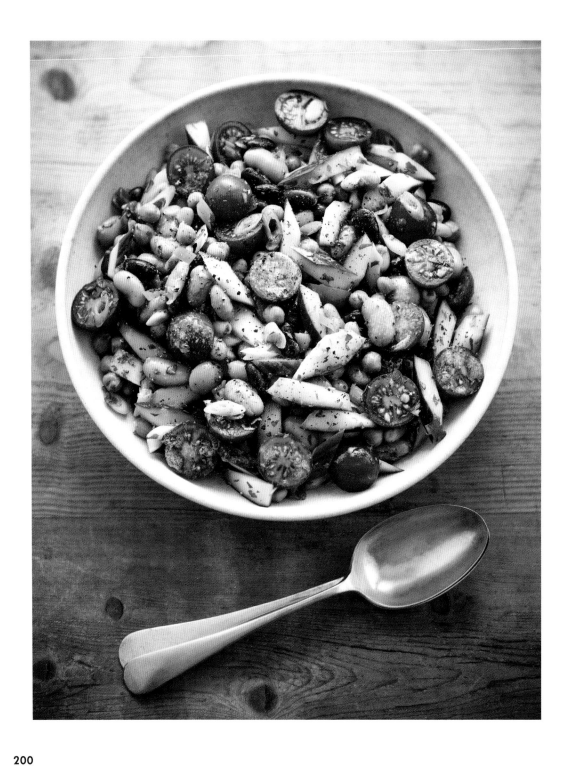

Day-trip bean salad

 Vegan

Serves 4 as a side

Takes 15 minutes

2 x 400g tins of mixed beans, drained and rinsed

1 cucumber, cut into chunks

150g cherry tomatoes, halved

1 bunch of spring onions, finely sliced

2 tablespoons finely chopped parsley

For the dressing

1 clove of garlic, peeled and finely grated

3 tablespoons extra virgin olive oil

1 tablespoon red wine vinegar or apple cider vinegar

1 teaspoon Dijon mustard

salt and black pepper

A day out in our family wouldn't be the same without this salad, which has been in our picnics as long as I can remember. The beans are wonderfully filling and sing out in their garlicky herb dressing. As you'll have guessed, this salad travels beautifully, but it's also ideal for a summer spread or as a simple meal eaten at home.

Tip the beans into a sieve or colander set over the sink and rinse for about 30 seconds under the cold tap, until the water draining off runs clear. Allow the beans to dry off a little so that they don't make the salad too wet.

Place all the salad ingredients, including the beans, in a large mixing bowl and toss to combine.

Whisk the ingredients for the dressing together in a small bowl, or use a clean jam jar to shake them together.

Pour the dressing over the salad and mix well to combine.

Super crunchy rainbow slaw

 Vegan

Serves 4 as a side

Takes 15 minutes

This is a side for numerous mains, including meat and fish, and it's always popular, whether served at a summer barbecue or a Boxing Day buffet. With its vibrant carrots, red cabbage, yellow peppers and green sugar snaps, this is a rainbow slaw with a crunch for all seasons.

3 carrots, peeled and julienned (cut into long thin batons)

50g red cabbage, thinly sliced with a knife or mandolin or using the grater function of a food processor

50g white cabbage, thinly sliced with a knife or mandolin or using the grater function of a food processor

50g sugar snaps, sliced lengthways

2 yellow peppers, deseeded and thinly sliced

2 spring onions, very thinly sliced (optional, depending on whether you like the taste)

3 tablespoons roughly chopped coriander

3 tablespoons mayonnaise (homemade (page 234) or shop-bought) Use an egg-free mayonnaise for a vegan option

1 teaspoon Dijon mustard

1 lemon, juice only (to taste)

1 tablespoon nigella seeds (optional)

salt and black pepper

Put all the veg into a mixing bowl and toss to combine.

Add the rest of the ingredients and mix everything together either with your hands or using a large spoon. Season, taste and add more lemon juice or black pepper if needed. Serve alongside meat or fish, top up a lunchbox, tuck in a lettuce wrap . . .

The slaw will keep in the fridge in a sealed container for up to 3 days.

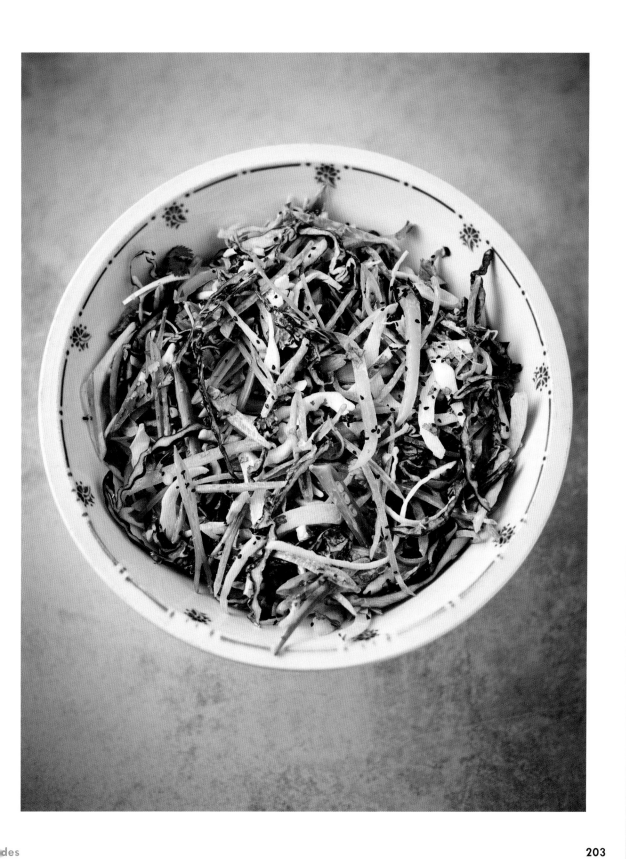

Roasted broccoli with chilli, almonds and pecorino

(if vegetarian pecorino or Parmesan used)

Serves 2 as a side

Takes 25 minutes

40g butter

1 tablespoon olive oil

1 head of broccoli, cut in half through the stem

1 red chilli, sliced (leave the seeds in if you like the heat)

50g almonds, crushed or flaked

60g pecorino cheese (or Parmesan)

Roasted broccoli with hot melted butter, toasted almond crunch, fiery chilli and a final flourish of salty pecorino to seal the deal – this is a deliciously bold side that shouts with flavour.

Preheat the oven to 180°C/160°C fan/gas 4.

Place a large oven-safe frying pan or casserole dish on a medium heat and melt the butter with the oil.

Put both broccoli halves into the pan, cut side down, and cook for 10 minutes. Use the melted butter to baste the broccoli regularly. If you run out of butter for basting, add a touch more butter to the pan.

Add the chilli and almonds and coat them in the butter, then put the whole pan into the oven and roast for around 10 minutes, until the broccoli is cooked through. If you pierce it with a skewer or a small sharp knife you will have little resistance.

Remove from the oven and cover with a generous handful of pecorino or Parmesan, which will slightly melt into the hot broccoli.

Serve while hot, or allow to cool and add to your lunchbox or salad.

Peperonata

Serves 4

Takes 1 hour 15 minutes

Hands-on: 15 minutes
Hands-off: 1 hour

4 tablespoons olive oil

1 onion, sliced

4 large peppers, red, yellow
and orange combination,
deseeded and roughly
chopped

5 cloves of garlic, peeled
and very thinly sliced

400g tin of chopped
tomatoes

2 tablespoons chopped basil
leaves

salt and black pepper

Jammy, slow-cooked peppers make peperonata a perfect accompaniment to a host of dishes – from a meat or fish side, to a salad topper or a cheeseboard chutney, this scarlet, sticky Italian classic is a winner every time.

Heat the olive oil in a saucepan over a medium heat and add the onion. Cook for around 5 minutes until starting to soften. Stir often to avoid the onion taking on any colour.

Add the peppers and garlic and continue to cook gently until they start to soften. This will probably take around 10 minutes.

Add the tomatoes, then turn the heat right down and cook for an hour at a gentle simmer until the peppers are soft right through and the tomato is rich and sticky. Stir occasionally to avoid the sauce catching on the bottom.

Remove from the heat, add the basil and season to taste. Leave to cool, then store in an airtight jar in the fridge until needed. It will keep for up to a week.

Marinated baked feta

Serves 2

Takes 20 minutes,
plus marinating time

200g feta

2 tablespoons extra virgin
  olive oil

5 thyme sprigs, leaves
  picked off

1 unwaxed lemon, zest only

½ teaspoon chilli flakes

20g pitted olives, halved

6 cherry tomatoes, halved

black pepper

The salty feta and olives, offset by the sweetness of the tomatoes, all cut through with the freshness of the lemon and thyme, make this dish a bit of a classic in our groups, especially as people grow in confidence with their cooking – adding more tomatoes here, a different fresh herb there. This recipe is a great example of owning your Full Diet food and making it perfectly right for you.

Line a small roasting tin with baking paper and put in the feta.

Whisk together the olive oil, thyme leaves, lemon zest, chilli flakes and some black pepper and pour all over the feta. Lift up the feta to make sure it is coated all over. Cover and leave to marinate in the fridge for a minimum of 2 hours but ideally overnight.

Preheat the oven to 200°C/180°C fan/gas 6.

Uncover the roasting tin, add the olives and cherry tomatoes, and place in the oven for 15–20 minutes, until the feta is baked through and golden brown at the edges.

This is delicious eaten straight from the oven as is, or along with steamed green beans, carrot and poppy seed crunch (page 223), crumbled into a salad, or enjoyed in a packed lunch or picnic.

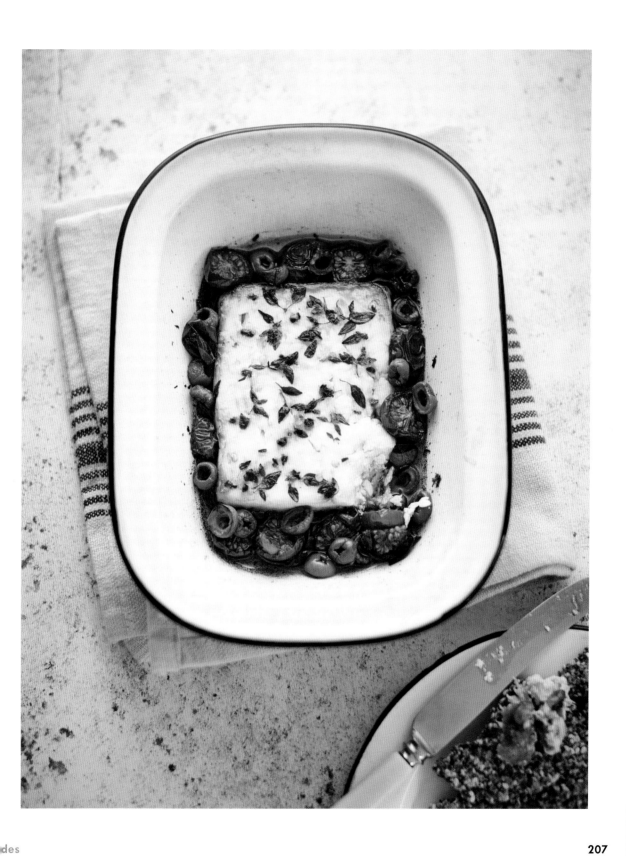

Beetroot gratin

**Serves 2 generously
or 4 as a side**

Takes 1 hour 15 minutes, plus
infusing and resting time

Hands-on: 15 minutes
Hands-off: 1 hour

350ml double cream

20g fresh thyme

4 cloves of garlic, peeled
and crushed

¼ teaspoon ground or
freshly grated nutmeg

500g bunch of beetroot

butter, for greasing

salt and black pepper

To serve

fresh soft herbs, such
as dill or tarragon

The earthy flavour of beetroot combined with the richness of the double cream makes this dish a star in its own right. Perfect as a side with red meat, chicken or fish, or serve a more generous portion to eat as a main meal.

Put the cream, thyme and garlic cloves into a saucepan and bring the cream to the boil. Immediately turn off the heat and allow the cream to cool back to room temperature – this will take around an hour.

Once the infused cream is at room temperature, pour it through a sieve into a mixing bowl. Discard the aromatics remaining in the sieve. Add the nutmeg and some seasoning to the cream and stir gently to combine.

If you'd like to avoid staining your hands, you can wear some disposable gloves or clean washing-up gloves for this step. Peel the beetroot, then, using either a mandolin or a very sharp knife, cut the beets into 2mm-thick rounds.

Preheat the oven to 200°C/180°C fan/gas 6. Grease a small ovenproof dish with butter; you want a dish approx. 20cm x 15cm x 6cm deep.

Lay the beetroot slices in the dish, making sure to overlap them only slightly as you want them all to be completely coated by the cream. Once they are all added, press them down gently using a spatula and then pour over the cream.

Place the dish on a baking sheet to catch any splashes and bake in the oven for 60 minutes.

Check the gratin after 45 minutes, as some ovens are hotter than others and it may be done. Remove from the oven and use the tip of a knife or a skewer to see if the beetroot is tender all the way through. You don't want any resistance. If it's not ready, return to the oven and cook for the full 60 minutes, then test again with a knife or skewer. If it is not done, return to the oven for a further 10 minutes or until soft.

Once cooked, allow to stand for at least 15 minutes for the cream to stop bubbling and the beets to settle, then garnish with the fresh herbs before serving.

Beetroot latkes

Serves 4 as a side

Takes 30 minutes

A delicious take on a popular favourite, these crispy beetroot latkes are wonderfully versatile. Pile them up with sour cream, or they're equally good topped with smoked salmon, cream cheese and a garnish of fresh chives.

500g beetroot, peeled and grated

1½ tablespoons ground flaxseed

1 tablespoon finely chopped chives

1 tablespoon finely chopped dill

black pepper

olive oil, for frying

To serve

8 teaspoons sour cream

4 hard-boiled eggs, peeled and halved

a pinch of chilli powder

salt and black pepper

Put the oven on a very low heat, to keep the latkes warm once you've made them.

Give the grated beetroot a good squeeze to lose some of the water content, then place it in a large mixing bowl. It can be a good idea to use a pair of clean rubber gloves or food prep gloves when cooking with beetroot, to avoid your hands becoming stained.

Add the flaxseed, herbs and black pepper to the beetroot and mix well.

Heat a large frying pan on a medium low heat and add just enough oil to coat the base.

Divide the beetroot mix into 8 and shape into rough patties. As you make each one, place it in the pan. Depending on the size of your pan, you may need to do two or three batches.

Gently press down on the top of each patty with a spatula to compress and flatten. Cook for 5–6 minutes, and once they are a deep golden and crisp on the edges, carefully turn the latkes over and cook for another 5–6 minutes on the other side.

Remove from the pan and blot the patties dry with kitchen paper to keep them crisp, then place in the oven to keep warm while you cook the remaining latkes.

Once you are ready to serve, top each latke with a little sour cream, half a boiled egg, a pinch of chilli powder and a little seasoning.

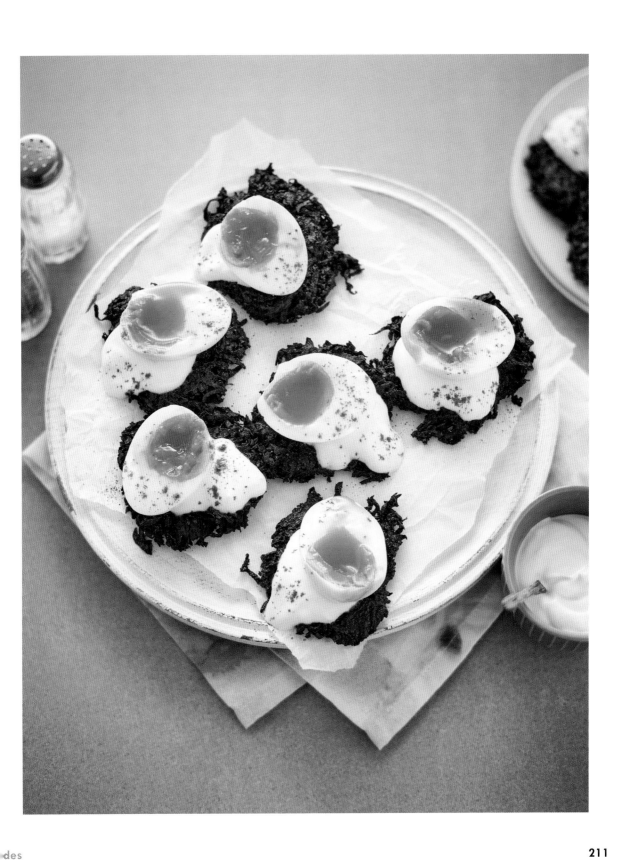

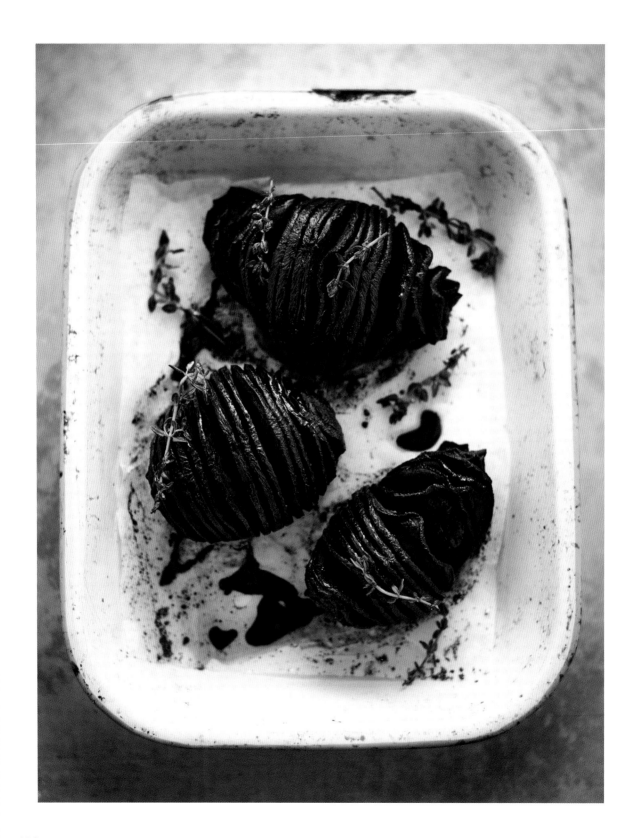

Hasselback(ish) beets

Serves 2 as a side

Takes 1 hour

Hands-on: 5 minutes
Hands-off: 55 minutes

3 medium beetroots, peeled
  and halved

1 tablespoon olive oil

¼ teaspoon garlic granules

1 teaspoon thyme leaves

salt and black pepper

The famed Swedish restaurant Hasselbacken, renowned for its fan-style potatoes, lends its name to these thin-sliced roasted beets. Crispy on the outside, soft and sweet on the inside, perfect as a meat or fish side, or served cold in a salad or on a cheeseboard.

Preheat the oven to 190°C/170°C fan/gas 5 and line a small roasting tin with baking paper.

Lay the beets cut side down on a chopping board in between two parallel wooden spoons. Use a sharp knife to slice every 5mm along the length of the beetroot, but not going all the way through – you want to stop around 5–10mm from the chopping board – the wooden spoons will prevent the knife going all the way down to the chopping board and will stop you cutting all the way through the beetroot. You'll finish with the beets intact, cut into a fan pattern.

Transfer the beets to the prepared roasting tin, drizzle over the olive oil, sprinkle over the garlic, and add the thyme and some seasoning. Roast in the oven for 50–60 minutes, until tender all the way through.

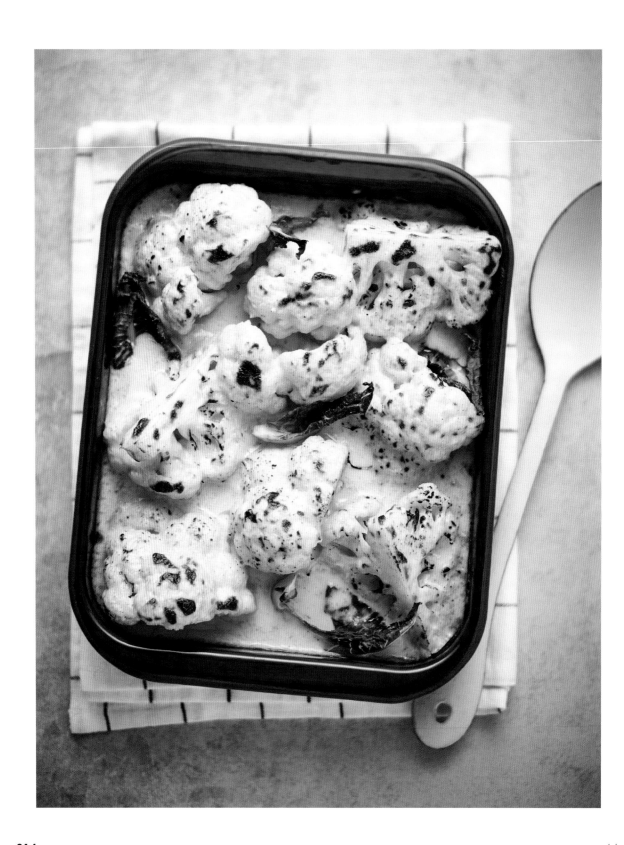

Cauliflower cheese wedges

**Serves 4 as a main
or 8 as a side**

Takes 45 minutes

Hands-on: 10 minutes
Hands-off: 30–35 minutes

2 cauliflowers, each cut into
 4 quarters, reserving the
 smaller leaves

50g butter

2 tablespoons arrowroot
 powder

½ teaspoon garlic powder

¼ teaspoon ground or
 freshly grated nutmeg

¼ teaspoon cayenne pepper

500ml whole milk

1 teaspoon Dijon mustard

200g Cheddar, grated

salt and black pepper

There is so much to love about these nutty wedges of cauliflower drenched in a rich creamy cheese sauce and baked until bubbling. Ideal as a side or (for fewer people) as a main served with a crisp green salad.

Set up a steamer and once the water is boiling, add the cauliflower wedges. Cook for 12 minutes, then remove from the heat.

While the cauliflower is steaming, preheat the oven to 200°C/180°C fan/gas 6 and get a non-stick roasting tin ready.

Heat the butter in a saucepan and add the arrowroot. Cook until the butter starts to smell a little bit nutty. Add the garlic powder, nutmeg and cayenne and stir to incorporate.

Slowly start to add the milk, about 50ml at a time, stirring well with each addition until all is combined. Cook for just a few minutes, until the sauce thickens. Stir in the Dijon mustard and remove from the heat. Add the grated Cheddar, season with salt and pepper and gently stir until melted.

Place the steamed cauliflower wedges in the roasting tin and pour over the sauce. Tuck in the cauliflower leaves and season with salt and pepper.

Bake in the oven for 25–30 minutes, until golden brown and bubbling.

Cauliflower rice

  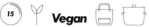

Serves 2 as a side

Takes 10 minutes

When I discuss rice with my patients, we almost always agree that what we appreciate is its sponge-like ability to absorb sauce – whether with a chilli, curry or stir-fry, it's the sauce rather than the rice that's the main event. It doesn't seem worthwhile to spike blood sugar levels when cauliflower rice can do an even better job delivering delicious sauce from plate to you. Aside from being a delicious bed for the sauce to seep into, cauliflower rice will keep your blood sugar level steady and your insulin levels low (fat-burning), while at the same time nourishing your gut bacteria with their own high-fibre meal.

300g cauliflower, cut into florets, stem discarded

15g butter or 1 tablespoon olive oil (for a vegan option)

salt and black pepper

Place the florets in the bowl of a food processor and whiz until you have a fine rice-like consistency. Alternatively, grate using the largest side of a box grater.

Heat a large frying pan on a high heat. Check the pan is hot enough by adding a handful of cauliflower – if it sizzles when it goes in, the pan is ready and you can add the rest of the cauliflower.

Leave the cauliflower for a minute, then turn it over with a spatula. Turn again after another 15 seconds. You want it to start taking on a little colour, but not burning. Keep it moving until it starts to smell nutty and has reduced in bulk, which happens when some of the water has evaporated off – this will help soften the cauliflower.

After about 4 minutes, add the butter (or oil if using), season and cook for another 2–3 minutes, by which time it should still have a little bite and taste nutty, like wholegrain rice. If you prefer it softer, continue cooking until it is done to your liking.

Cauliflower mash

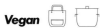 **Vegan**

Serves 2 as a side

Takes 15–20 minutes

This is a bowl of fluffy, golden goodness. It's ideal as a side, a soft bed for a curry or Bolognese, or as a topping on a fish or shepherd's pie. Or you could enjoy it as the main event, with a handful of Cheddar cheese melted into the hot, creamy mash, stirred through with freshly ground black pepper and served immediately.

400g cauliflower, roughly chopped into florets

40g butter or 3 tablespoons olive oil (for a vegan option)

salt and black pepper

Optional extras (works best to choose one at a time)

garlic powder

ground or freshly grated nutmeg

green herbs, such as parsley or tarragon

Cheddar cheese

cream cheese

Place a saucepan of salted water on a medium high heat. Once boiling, add the cauliflower and boil for around 6–8 minutes, until very tender and easy to pierce with the tip of a knife. Drain in a colander and allow to steam dry for a minute or two in the colander — you don't want any excess water in the mash.

Transfer the cauliflower to a food processor and add the butter (or olive oil if using). Alternatively you can place the cauliflower and butter (or oil if using) in a large bowl and use a stick blender. Blitz for a couple of minutes, until totally smooth.

Season generously and blitz once more.

Add any optional extra of your choosing.

Green dream broccoli mash

  Vegan

Serves 2 as a side

Takes 15 minutes

1 head of broccoli, cut into florets, stalk diced

1 clove of garlic, peeled and finely grated

¼ teaspoon ground or freshly grated nutmeg

40g butter or 3 tablespoons olive oil (for a vegan option)

1–2 tablespoons grated Cheddar, Gruyère or Parmesan (optional)

salt and black pepper

The butter, garlic and nutmeg elevate the broccoli into a gloriously smooth green dream. This is a super versatile side and works brilliantly with a wealth of other dishes, including many meat and fish recipes. For an extra tasty, rich depth of flavour, grate in some cheese at the last minute, to melt into the hot mash.

Bring a large pan of salted water up to the boil and add the broccoli. Cook for 4–6 minutes, until it is tender all the way through. Drain in a colander and return to the pan. Put the pan back on the heat and continue cooking for just long enough to remove any excess water.

Add the garlic, nutmeg and butter, then mash with a potato masher or blitz with a stick blender or in a food processor. You can leave it slightly chunky or keep working it into a smoother mash, depending on your preference.

Season to taste and stir in the grated cheese (if using).

side

Celeriac mash

Serves 2 as a side

Takes 25 minutes

This is a delicious low-sugar alternative to mashed potato. You can thicken it up by adding half a tin of drained butter beans to the water while boiling the celeriac, then mashing. Or you can make it extra rich and creamy by adding a couple of spoons of crème fraîche while mashing. Finally you can add an extra burst of flavour by stirring in some freshly chopped herbs like thyme or parsley just before serving.

1 celeriac, peeled and cubed

40g butter or 3 tablespoons olive oil (for a vegan option)

salt and black pepper

Optional – check recipe introduction for how to use

200g butter beans, drained and rinsed

2 tablespoons fresh herbs, such as thyme or parsley

2 tablespoons crème fraîche

Put the celeriac into a pan of salted water and cook for around 20 minutes, or until the cubes are soft all the way through when pierced with the tip of a sharp knife.

Drain the celeriac in a colander and put back into the hot saucepan. Place the pan back on the heat for a minute or two, to evaporate any excess water before mashing.

Take off the heat, add the butter (or olive oil if using) and some seasoning, and mash well. You can use a potato masher or a stick blender. Alternatively, transfer the celeriac to a food processor, add the butter and seasoning and blitz to a smooth mash.

Celeriac chips

 Vegan

Serves 2 as a side

Takes 50 minutes

Hands-on: 5 minutes
Hands-off: 50 minutes

Celeriac is gorgeous in its own right but also a wonderfully versatile alternative to potatoes. These chips have all the texture and salty crunch of potato chips but none of the blood sugar surge. Delicious with a 'good stuff' cheeseburger (page 105) or to eat as 'fish and chips' with any fish recipe. You can also cut them slightly larger, to serve as Full Diet roasties with your Sunday lunch.

1 celeriac

2 tablespoons olive oil

1 teaspoon paprika

salt and black pepper

Heat the oven to 200°C/180°C fan/gas 6 and line a baking tray with non-stick baking paper.

Peel the celeriac and cut it into 1.5cm chips (you will need a large sharp knife, as the skin can be thick and a bit unyielding – it will also make cutting the chips much easier).

Place the chips on the baking tray, add the olive oil, paprika and seasoning and toss everything to coat. Place in the hot oven for 30 minutes, then remove, shake the tray to turn the chips, and return to the oven for another 15–20 minutes, until the celeriac is tender and cooked through.

Roast Brussels sprouts

Serves 2 as a side

Takes approx. 30–40 minutes

Hands-on: 5–10 minutes
Hands-off: 30 minutes

200g Brussels sprouts, trimmed
and each sliced in half

65g diced pancetta

1 red chilli, cut in half and
sliced thinly (leave the seeds
in if you like the heat)

1 tablespoon olive oil

50g flaked almonds

1 unwaxed lemon, zest only

salt and black pepper

Packed with fibre and phytonutrients, sprouts are loved by your gut bacteria. Roasted with pancetta and almonds, with a fiery chilli kick and finished with a lemon zest zing, these roasted sprouts are delicious as a side or added to salads, and, of course, ideal for your Christmas-lunch table.

Preheat the oven to 200°C/180°C fan/gas 6 and line a roasting tin with baking paper.

Place the sprouts, pancetta and chilli in the tin and gently toss to combine. Drizzle over the olive oil and season with a little salt and pepper.

Put the tin into the oven and cook for 15 minutes. Remove, add the almonds and stir, then put back into the oven for another 15 minutes. If everything is looking golden and the sprouts are tender, remove from the oven. If not, return for another 10 minutes (or until done to your liking).

Grate over the lemon zest and toss everything together before serving.

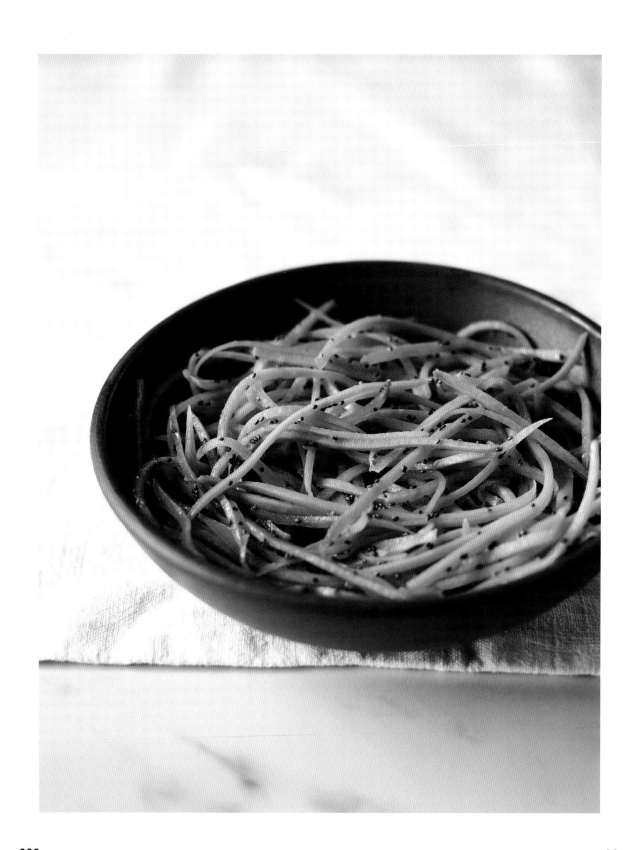

Carrot and poppy seed crunch

 Vegan

Serves 2 as a side

Takes 5 minutes

2 large carrots, peeled and julienned (finely sliced into long thin batons)

1 tablespoon extra virgin olive oil

½ lemon, juice only

1 tablespoon poppy seeds

salt and black pepper

This sweet and crunchy side adds a joyful splash of colourful flavour to your meal. It's a recipe you'll get a lot of mileage out of – perfect at home to accompany main dishes, and also ideal for lunchboxes, picnics and barbecues.

Place all the ingredients except the salt in a mixing bowl (if the salt is added prior to serving, it will make the carrot go limp and watery). Use your hands to gently mix everything together, then store in the fridge until needed.

When you are ready to serve, add a pinch of salt, stir to combine, taste and add more lemon juice and/or salt and black pepper if needed.

essentials and drinks

I hope that this section will be the beginning of your own Full Diet Essentials collection. It's here that I want to start you off with some drinks, condiments and dressings so that you can build on these ideas with your own additions as you get into your Programme stride.

Shop-bought condiments and dressings tend to come with either a lot of added sugar, dubious ingredients, or both. This is why I've included recipes for popular condiments like ketchup (page 236) and versatile dressings such as tangy salad dressing (page 232) and creamy salad dressing (page 233) which will perfectly complement a glorious array of your delicious Full Diet recipes. This is not to say that these foods when shop-bought are off-Programme, more that it gives you options to either make your own at home or to buy pre-prepared if you can find versions with straightforward ingredients and no added sugar.

I am frequently asked by my patients what drinks work well on the Programme. You can see in the 'Choose to Eat' list on pages 242–5 that still and sparkling water, coffee, tea, and herbal and fruit teas are all part of The Full Diet, but sometimes you might want an extra-cooling drink or an invigorating seltzer. It's here that refreshing options like the cool cucumber and basil infusion (page 240) or pomegranate and apple refresher (page 241) really come into their own. And of course do draw on these recipes and ideas to create other flavour combinations that are perfectly right and refreshing for you.

Crunchy kale crisps

 Vegan

Serves 4

Takes 40–45 minutes

Hands-on: 10–15 minutes
Hands-off: 30 minutes

250g kale

1 tablespoon extra virgin
  olive oil

sea salt and black pepper

Optional additional flavours

½ teaspoon paprika or
  garlic granules or cumin

If you thought that crisps have to be ultra-processed, think again. These kale crisps are full of vegetable goodness: no tricks, no dubious ingredients. They are great served at parties or eaten as a snack. They travel well in a lunchbox and add an extra green salty crunch as a salad topper.

Preheat the oven to 150°C/130°C fan/gas 2 and line two baking trays with non-stick baking paper.

Remove the tough stems from the kale and tear the leaves into similar sized pieces – you don't want the pieces too small, as they do shrink quite a lot in the oven.

Put the kale into a mixing bowl and add the oil. Mix the kale and oil together well with your hands – you want all the kale to be coated and to slightly break it down.

Tip the kale on to the two baking trays and spread out in a thin layer, trying to prevent anything overlapping. Place in the oven for 15 minutes, then remove, turn, and bake for another 15 minutes.

Remove the trays from the oven and take out any kale that is crispy and done, then return the trays to the oven in 5-minute intervals, removing the kale that has gone crispy each time until all the crisps are done.

Sprinkle with sea salt and black pepper, allow to completely cool, then store in an airtight container in a cool place for 2 or 3 days.

If you are using a flavour, such as paprika, garlic or cumin, add when mixing the kale with the oil before it goes into the oven.

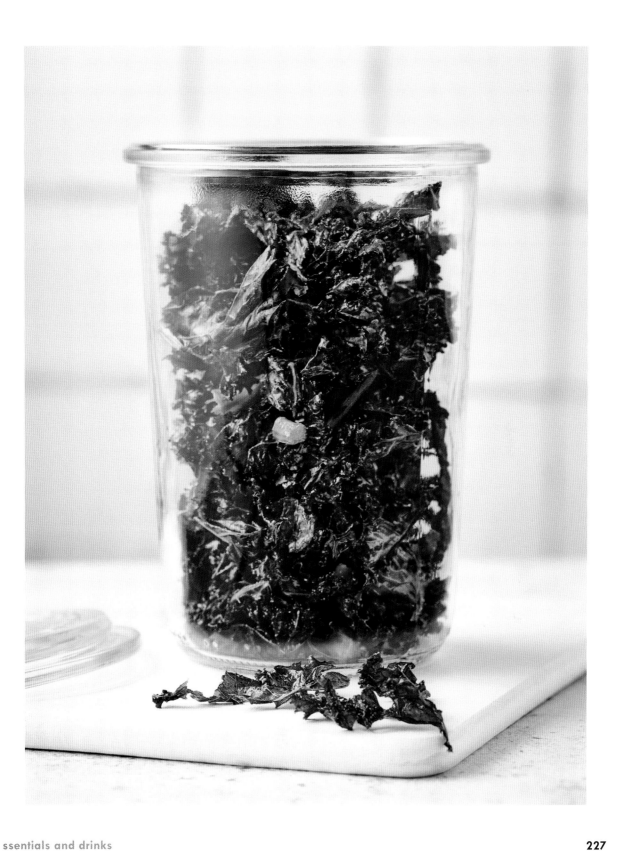

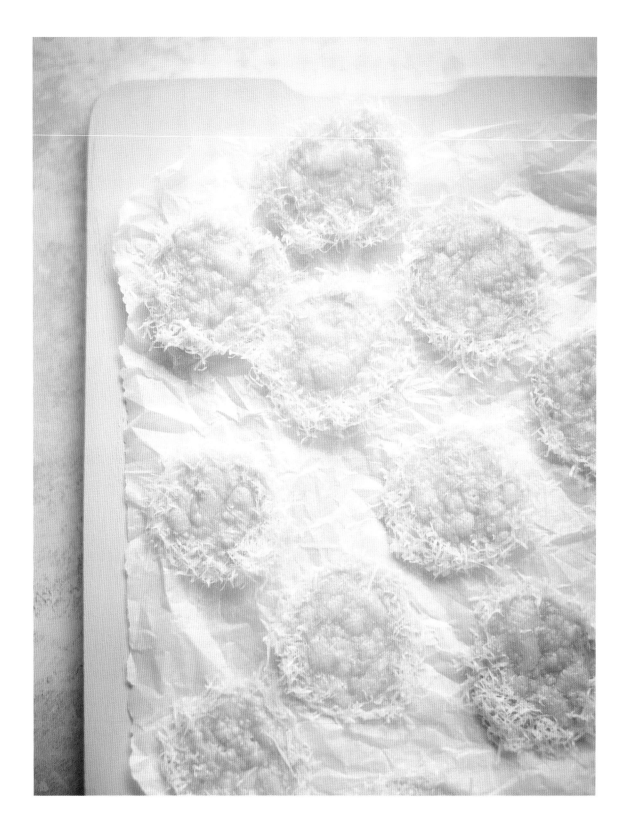

Parmesan crisps

15

(if vegetarian
Parmesan used)

Makes 4 servings

Takes 10–15 minutes

160g Pamesan, grated

black pepper

The ultimate salty crunch – serve before a meal if you have guests, brilliant as a snack, or crumble over a green salad for that extra Parmesan umami lift.

Preheat the oven to 180°C/160°C fan/gas 4. Line two baking sheets with non-stick baking paper (the non-stick is very important).

Place the grated Parmesan in small mounds on the baking sheet and pat each mound down into a disc shape. You want a thin but even layer without any holes (or it won't stick together). You don't need to press it down, but ideally it's about 2mm thick all over. Grind a little black pepper over each one.

Carefully put the trays into the oven. The cheese will collapse and melt and join – that's OK, as you can break it into crisps when it cools.

Remove the trays from the oven once the crisps are going a deep golden brown around the edges and the middle is bubbling away. This could be anywhere from 3 to 10 minutes depending on the size and thickness of your crisps, so keep a close eye.

Leave to cool on the trays for 10 minutes, then slide the baking paper off the hot trays. Allow to cool fully before lifting off the paper. Break into crisp-size pieces.

The crisps can be stored in an airtight container in a cool place for 2 to 3 days.

Super seeded crackers

 Vegan

Makes 4–6 servings (depending on how you're using them)

Takes 1 hour 10 minutes

Hands-on: 10 minutes
Hands-off: 1 hour

150g ground flaxseed, sunflower and pumpkin seed mix (Linwoods is a good brand for this)

50g ground flaxseed

50g sesame seeds

30g poppy seeds

180–210ml water

salt

black pepper (optional)

From loading up with hummus or guacamole, to dipping into an oozing, golden egg yolk, crumbling into a soup or salad, or stacked high on a cheeseboard, these versatile crackers are true Full Diet all-rounders. The delicious mixture of fibre-rich seeds makes these a great option for your gut bacteria too. If you like, you can make a large batch by doubling the quantities – they will keep in a sealed container for up to a week.

Preheat the oven to 170°C/150°C fan/gas 3 and get two large sheets of non-stick baking paper and a rolling pin ready.

Place all the ingredients aside from the water in a large mixing bowl.

Add as much of the water as you need to just bring it all together into a shapeable paste, then leave to sit for 5 minutes.

Turn out the mix on to one of the sheets of baking paper. Place the other sheet on top and press with your hands, then use the rolling pin to get the mix as thin as possible. Use a spatula or something with a straight edge to tidy up the edges of the seed mix. The shape you roll the mix out to needs to be compatible with your baking tray – you should be able to get it on the one tray, but you might need two.

Once you have the mix around 2–3mm thick, remove the top sheet of paper and slide the rolled out seeds on top of the bottom sheet of baking paper on to the baking tray.

Place in the oven for 30 minutes, then turn the tray 180 degrees and cook the mix for another 20–30 minutes, until dry and crisp with no squishy bit in the middle if you push down gently.

Remove from the oven and allow to cool on the tray. Once completely cool, peel the crackers off the baking paper and snap into whatever shape and size you would like them to be. Store in an airtight container.

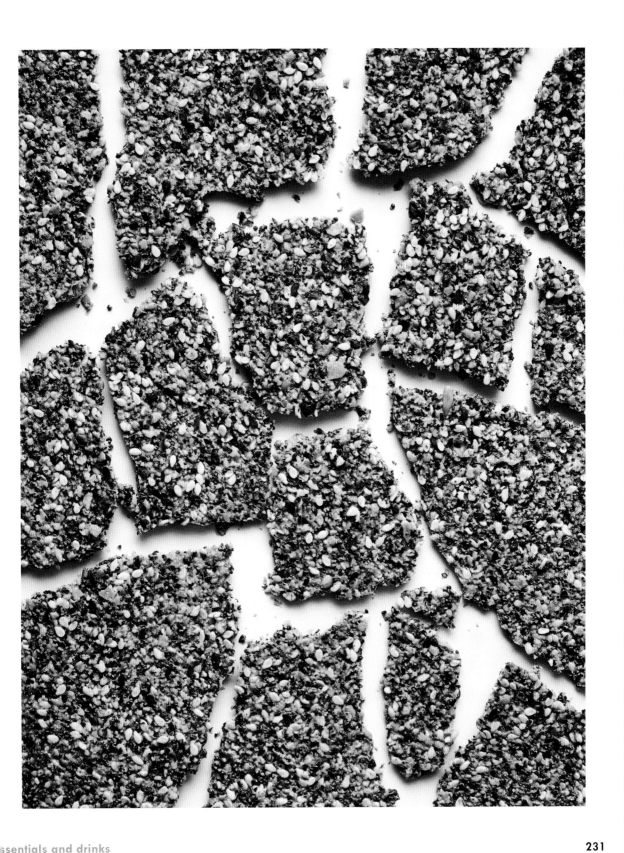

Tangy salad dressing

 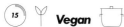

Serves 2–4

Takes 5 minutes

3 tablespoons extra virgin olive oil

1 unwaxed lime, zest and juice

1 teaspoon oregano (fresh or dried)

¼ teaspoon chilli flakes (optional)

salt and black pepper

A burst of citrus lime tang adds a fresh twist to salads. You can also add some heat with some chilli flakes for an extra fiery kick.

Place all the ingredients in a clean jam jar and shake to combine. Check the seasoning and adjust to taste. Store any leftovers in the fridge in the jam jar for another day.

Creamy salad dressing

Serves 2–4

Takes 5 minutes

2 tablespoons mayonnaise
(homemade (page 234)
or shop-bought)

2 tablespoons full-fat Greek
yoghurt

1 unwaxed lemon, zest
and juice

1 clove of garlic, peeled
and finely grated

1 tablespoon chopped fresh
herbs, such as parsley

salt and black pepper

A velvety rich dressing, perfect on a green leaf, tomato, cucumber or mixed salad – or anything else you want to use it with. Infinitely fresher and tastier than anything made by the food industry – this is dressing as it should be.

Put all the ingredients into a clean jam jar and shake to combine.

Check the seasoning and adjust to taste.

Use as needed and store the rest in a sealed jam jar in the fridge for up to 3 days.

Mayonnaise

Makes approx. 280g

Takes 10 minutes

You will find this homemade mayonnaise is completely different from shop-bought versions. Rich with olive oil and eggs, perfectly balanced by the essential acidity and freshness of the lemon — from mashing into a simple egg mayo to a delicious accompaniment to meat, fish, vegetables and beyond, this mayonnaise is so beautifully versatile that it may well become one of your Full Diet go-to classic recipes.

2 egg yolks

1 teaspoon white wine vinegar

1 teaspoon Dijon mustard

1 teaspoon cold water

250ml light olive oil (light means light in both colour and flavour, not low fat)

1–2 teaspoons freshly squeezed lemon juice

salt and black pepper

Place the egg yolks, vinegar, mustard, water and a small pinch of salt in a mini chopper or the small bowl of a food processor and start the motor running. Slowly but consistently drizzle in the olive oil.

When you have poured in about half the oil, add 1 teaspoon of lemon juice and continue slowly pouring in the oil.

Keep the motor running until all the oil is combined and your mayonnaise is beautifully glossy and thick. Check the taste and adjust the seasoning if needed, then add a little more lemon juice to your preferred taste.

Spoon into an airtight jar and store in the fridge for up to 2 weeks.

Apple sauce

Serves 4–6

Takes 20 minutes

This apple sauce is a tasty, sweet accompaniment to pork dishes. It can be enjoyed warm from the pan or cooked in advance and used when needed. It also makes a delicious compote, perfect as a topping to full-fat Greek yoghurt.

4 Bramley apples, peeled, cored and diced

50g butter

a pinch of mixed spice

Put the apples and butter into a saucepan and place on a low heat. Cook the apples gently in the melted butter, stirring until the fruit just starts to break down. This will take around 15 minutes.

Add the mixed spice.

Stir more vigorously for another 5 minutes so you end up with a much smoother purée. Then turn off the heat and either serve warm, or allow to cool, then store in a clean jam jar in the fridge for up to 5 days.

Fresh homemade ketchup

 Vegan

Makes approx. 800ml

Takes 1 hour,
plus cooling time

Hands-on: 10 minutes
Hands-off: 50 minutes

Ketchup is a perennially loved condiment because of the sweet umami yum that it adds to countless savoury dishes. Shop-bought ketchups often contain so much added sugar that they give a meal an almost dessert-like quality. The Full Diet fresh homemade ketchup is entirely different – containing only the natural sweetness of the tomatoes, it still retains that same magic of offsetting a wealth of mains while keeping your blood sugar beautifully stable. Pass the ketchup, please!

1kg ripe tomatoes, cut into even chunks

6 cloves of garlic, peeled

3 tablespoons extra virgin olive oil

1 tablespoon red wine vinegar or apple cider vinegar

1 tablespoon mixed herbs

2 teaspoons dried oregano

½ teaspoon onion powder

¼ teaspoon ground or freshly grated nutmeg

¼ teaspoon ground cinnamon

100g tomato purée

salt and black pepper

Preheat the oven to 200°C/180°C fan/gas 6 and line a large roasting tin with baking paper.

Add the tomatoes and all the other ingredients except the tomato purée. Stir well to mix and coat everything. Level things out, then put the tray into the oven for 30 minutes.

Remove from the oven and stir in the tomato purée. Cook for another 20 minutes, then remove and allow to cool for at least 30 minutes.

Transfer everything to a food processor and blitz until smooth. Let the motor run for at least 3–4 minutes. Alternatively, you can use a stick blender.

Set up a large jug with a sieve over it and pour the sauce through the sieve. Gently coax the sauce through the sieve with a wooden spoon into the jug below. Check the taste and adjust the seasoning if needed.

You now have a batch of ketchup ready for bottling. Use a clean sterilized bottle (an old passata bottle is ideal).

Store in the fridge for up to 2 weeks.

Pow-pow! chilli sauce

 Vegan

Makes 250g

Takes 5 minutes if you have already made the ketchup

200ml homemade ketchup (page 236)

1 teaspoon olive oil

5 red chillies, each cut into 3 or 4 pieces (either deseeded or seeds left in if you like the extra heat)

This fiery chilli sauce is a taste sensation knockout. Perfect for adding that extra kick whenever you are looking for even more chilli heat. From your 'good stuff' cheeseburger to your Full avo-salsa burrito, this fiery chilli sauce is a taste sensation knock-out. Pow-pow!

Place the ketchup in a mini chopper or in a container suitable for use with a stick blender.

Heat the olive oil in a small frying pan and add the chillies. If you like it really hot you can mix up the types of chillies, for example using Scotch bonnet or Thai chillies, varying the number of chillies, and so on.

Cook the chillies on a high heat until the skin starts to go a dark golden brown. This shouldn't take more than 3–4 minutes. Take care as the fumes from the chillies can be quite strong. Remove from the heat and add the chillies to the ketchup.

Blitz all together and leave to cool, then transfer to an airtight tub or bottle and store in the fridge, where it will keep for up to a week.

Herbal ice tea

 Vegan

Makes 1 litre

Takes 5 minutes,
plus cooling and
chilling time

3 herbal tea bags of one
variety (examples include
lemongrass and ginger, or
ginger, or chamomile, or
rooibos, or nettle)

1 unwaxed lemon

sprig of fresh mint (optional)

If you have herbal teabags in the cupboard and are looking for another way to use them – this is your answer. Choose flavours you enjoy and experiment, depending on the tea you have available. Rather than using them in a hot drink, try allowing them to infuse, then chilling and serving cold over ice, to give a whole new taste experience.

Boil the kettle, then pour 1 litre of boiling water into a large heatproof jug and add the teabags.

Allow to brew for 3–5 minutes, depending on how strong you like the flavour from the bag.

Remove the teabags and squeeze the juice of half a lemon into the jug. Slice the other half of the lemon and add to the jug. Add a sprig of fresh mint (if using). Stir well.

Set aside and allow the drink to cool, then chill in the fridge.

Serve over lots of ice. This keeps well in the fridge for a few days.

Ginger and lemon toddy

 Vegan

Makes 1 litre

Takes 5 minutes,
plus cooling and
chilling time

4 slices of fresh ginger
(around 1cm piece)

½ unwaxed lemon, cut into
2 wedges

This is a standout combination of fiery ginger with a refreshing lemon kick. Ideal as a revitalizing thirst-quencher at any time, or a non-alcoholic evening cocktail (one of my patients once compared the pep of the ginger to a shot of whisky – I'll leave you to be the judge of that!).

Boil a litre of water and pour it into a heatproof jug.

Peel the ginger and cut it into 4 slices, then add to the water. Squeeze the juice from the lemon wedges into the water, then add the lemon wedges to the jug as well. Stir well and allow to cool to room temperature, then put into the fridge to chill.

Store in the fridge until needed – it will keep for a couple of days. While you'll get a subtle taste almost immediately, the longer you leave it the deeper and more fiery the flavour from the ginger.

When serving, pour into a glass over a few ice cubes.

Cool cucumber and basil infusion

 Vegan

Makes 1 litre

Takes 5 minutes,
plus chilling time

1 litre water (still or
  sparkling), fridge cold

½ cucumber, peeled
  into ribbons

20 basil leaves

To serve

ice

The clean freshness of the cucumber infused with the sweet pungent basil leaves gives this cooling drink a refreshing depth of flavour. Carry it in a water bottle to perk up your on-the-go hydration, or make with sparkling water to serve as a stylish seltzer with meals or at a summer party.

Pour the water into a large jug (or two) and add the cucumber ribbons and basil leaves. Give everything a vigorous stir and allow to infuse in the fridge for at least 2 hours.

Serve over lots of ice for a really refreshing drink.

Grapefruit and soda quencher

 Vegan

Serves 1

Takes 2 minutes

350ml soda water,
  fridge cold

½ pink grapefruit

5 basil leaves

The perfect drink for a hot day, refreshing and zingy with a beautiful rose tinge. Increase the quantities as needed if enjoying with family and friends.

Cut a grapefruit in half. Cut one 5mm thick slice off the half you are using, cut the slice in half, and put both halves into a tall glass along with the basil leaves and some ice cubes.

Squeeze the remainder of the grapefruit half for its juice and pour over the ice. Add the cold soda water, stir well, and enjoy a really refreshing thirst-quencher.

Pomegranate and apple refresher

 Vegan

Makes 1 litre

Takes 5 minutes,
plus chilling time

1 litre water (still or sparkling)

50g pomegranate seeds
(from ½ medium-sized
pomegranate), lightly
crushed

1 small apple, cored
and sliced

This infusion, with its beautiful pink blush, is a refreshing blend of fresh sweet apple, perfectly balanced by the tart jewelled pomegranate seeds. Ideal to sip throughout the day at home, or to be carried in a bottle on the go for the times when you want a hydration boost that tastes as good as it looks.

Mix all the ingredients together in a large jug and leave in the fridge for a couple of hours to infuse. Serve poured over ice cubes, with some of the pomegranate seeds and apple in each glass.

This will keep in the fridge for a few days.

in full colour

your complete guide to eating on The Full Diet

Food lists

The Choose to Eat list

The eating principles of The Full Diet are based on the following food lists. As I do with my patients, I am going to ask you to pay most attention to the 'Choose to Eat' list, which is the reason I have put it first. Rather than focusing on missing foods that you are choosing not to eat (page 246), that were impacting your health and preventing you from being the weight you want to be, you can instead use your energy and enthusiasm to really get into the foods you *are* choosing to eat.

It is this mindset of putting the 'Choose to Eat' list front and centre that has led my patients to lose as much weight as people who have had gastric band surgery, while at the same time reversing health conditions and feeling good.

All the recipes in this book are based on this 'Choose to Eat' list. As you read the recipes, enjoy the beautiful photographs and take pride and pleasure in the incredible food you cook, I hope you will find, just as my patients have, that this is a delicious, joyful, life-enhancing way of eating.

Choose to eat:

Fruit and vegetables

- All vegetables (except for potatoes and other starchy vegetables, such as parsnips and sweet potatoes)
- Vegetables (can be fresh or frozen) – examples include: baby corn, broccoli, Brussels sprouts, cabbage, carrots, cauliflower, celeriac, garlic, green or runner beans, kale, mushrooms, onions and spinach
- Salad veg, such as celery, cucumber, radishes, lettuce and other green salad leaves

- Fruit-like vegetables, including avocados, aubergines, courgettes, peppers and tomatoes
- Lemons and limes
- Low- and medium-sugar fruit, such as apples, pears, blueberries, raspberries and strawberries (fruit is naturally sweet and contains sugar, so it's best not to overdo it – you could, for example, choose an apple one day, a handful of berries the next)

Eggs

Dairy

- Whole, full-fat milk (up to 100ml or so per day)
- Natural (plain) or Greek full-fat yoghurt (up to about 200g per day)
- Kefir (check it only has two ingredients – milk and beneficial bacteria cultures)
- Cheese, such as Cheddar, feta, halloumi, mozzarella, Parmesan and cream cheese (about 100g per day)
- Cream – single, double or clotted (about 2 tablespoons per day)
- Crème fraîche – full-fat (about 2 tablespoons per day)
- Butter – salted or unsalted, depending on your preference
- Non-dairy milk alternatives (check the ingredients are straightforward, for example, almond milk should contain only almonds, water and sometimes sea salt)

Meat

- Any kind of fresh meat – for example, beef, chicken, lamb, pork and turkey (check there's no breading, sauces or dubious ingredients and that it's just a one-ingredient food – meat!)
- Sausages – pork, beef, chicken or lamb with a high meat content, which means more than 90% meat
- Sliced cold cuts such as ham, chicken or turkey (check there's no added sugar, honey, syrups or breading)

Fish

- Any fish or shellfish, fresh or frozen (but not in breading, batter or sauces; it should be just one ingredient – fish!)

General

- Dips, such as hummus, tzatziki and guacamole
- Pesto
- Full-fat mayonnaise (check that the ingredients are straightforward and sound like food)
- Tabasco Original Red Pepper Hot Sauce
- Mustard
- Vinegar, such as white wine vinegar or apple cider vinegar
- Olives
- Tofu
- Cooking fats – olive oil, lard, coconut oil and ghee
- Fresh and dried herbs and spices
- Raw unsalted nuts, including almonds, Brazil nuts, macadamias, pecans, pistachios and walnuts (about a handful per day – check there are no added ingredients, such as a honey glaze)
- Nut butters, such as peanut butter and almond butter (about 2 teaspoons per day – check there is no added sugar)
- Seeds, such as flaxseed (also known as linseed), hemp seeds, pumpkin seeds, sesame seeds and sunflower seeds (a handful or two per day)
- Legumes, including lentils, beans (not baked beans) and chickpeas (up to one serving per day)
- Long-life tomato foods, like passata, tomato purée, tinned tomatoes and sun-dried tomatoes
- Good-quality dark chocolate – 85% or 90% cocoa solids
- Water – still or sparkling (but not flavoured or sweetened waters)
- Herbal or fruit tea – for example, camomile or mint

- Coffee – not with lots of milk (avoid a latte or flat white and please don't add syrups or sugar)
- Tea, including green tea (again, no added sugar)

The Choose Not to Eat list

When you digest these foods, they are broken down into sugar, which ends up in your blood. Your body then produces the hormone insulin (the fat controller). Insulin sweeps the sugar out of your blood and some of the sugar will be swept into fat storage. The foods on this list therefore make us very efficient at storing fat and so we put on weight.

Many of the foods on this list are also ultra-processed, which means they are usually high in sugar, low in fibre and full of odd substances, which not only drive overeating and weight gain but are likely to be related to other health problems too. The highly processed ingredients found in many of these foods, such as synthetic proteins, dyes and bulking agents, are not the right fuel for your brilliant body. From better-quality sleep and a brighter mood, to clear thinking and having more energy, my patients very quickly notice, and I'm sure you will too, how much better they feel when they ditch this sort of food.

At first, you might think this looks like a long list. In fact, these foods are mostly various combinations of the same few ingredients, like sugar (or ingredients quickly broken down into sugar), artificial sweeteners, synthetic fats and other dubious ingredients. Over the last forty years, the modern diet has come to be based on these foods. From weight gain to diabetes, fatigue and just not feeling well, it's a way of eating that's not working for most of us. For all these reasons, these are the foods I'd advise that you steer clear of:

Choose not to eat:

- Bread of any kind, including sliced, bagels, baguettes, chapatti, ciabatta, flatbreads, naan, pitta, rolls, tortillas and wraps
- Pasta
- Rice
- Couscous
- Noodles
- Breakfast cereals, including oats/porridge, muesli and granola
- Cereal bars
- Crackers
- Potatoes, including crisps and chips
- Baked goods, including biscuits, brownies, cakes, croissants, flapjacks, muffins and pastries
- Pizza
- Pastry (sweet or savoury)
- Sweets and chocolates
- Ice cream, sorbets and ice lollies
- Jam, marmalade and other sugar-based spreads
- Sugar, honey and syrups
- Artificial sweeteners
- High-sugar fruits, such as bananas, mangoes, grapes and pineapple
- Dried fruit
- Fruit juice (no matter how healthy the labelling claims)
- Smoothies (shop-bought or homemade)
- Squash drinks
- Fizzy drinks (including diet or no-calorie versions)
- Ketchup and other high-sugar condiments, such as barbecue sauce
- Shop-bought salad dressings
- Shop-bought sauces and stir-in cooking sauces
- Ready meals

What might my eating look like?

There are over 100 recipes in this book. To help with your meal planning, I have suggested what a couple of weeks on The Full Diet might look like. There are also 55 more recipes in *The Full Diet* book, so do include these too, as well as any others in your own cooking repertoire that fit the bill.

When you are up and running with your Eating Window, you're likely to find, as my patients do, that eating twice a day, sometimes with a snack in between, feels like the right amount of food in the eight-hour period. This is why I have written the Sample Meal Planner as two meals a day, but do take the traditional three meals approach if this feels right within your own Eating Window.

In the Meal Planners, I haven't made any assumptions about when in the day you prefer to spend more or less time on meal prep. Bigger ticket recipes are mentioned at different times of day, but you can decide when these suit you best. For example, some people prefer to have these sort of dishes in the evening, because that's when they have more time to cook, and this might also be your social meal of the day if you live with other people.

After some of the meals, I've included something for afters, but there's no particular reason behind why this follows some meals and not others. See what you feel like at the time and if you do want something else, like a bit of rich dark chocolate or some fruit with thick Greek yoghurt, then go for it and enjoy.

These Sample Meal Planners are just a guide. Please don't feel that you need to follow them precisely — or even follow them at all. One of the beautiful things about The Full Diet is its flexibility, so do have a look for reference, and then make eating plans that fit with your own Full Diet recipe and food preferences. This is your way of eating, so choose what feels best for you and all the Programme weight loss and health benefits will naturally follow.

Sample Meal Planner 1

	Monday	Tuesday	Wednesday
First meal of the day – the time that you open your Eating Window	Spiced tofu scramble (page 129)	Halloumi and veg traybake (page 138) A few squares of 85% or 90% dark chocolate – about the size of a credit card – with a mug of mint tea	The Full Caesar (page 63) Sliced pear with a handful of walnuts
Second meal	Fiery salmon and broccoli traybake (page 121) Strawberries and cream	Chicken tagine (page 91) with celeriac mash (page 219)	The 'good stuff' cheeseburger (page 105) with celeriac chips (page 220)
Snack	Vegetable crudités with 1 or 2 boiled eggs mashed up with mayonnaise or a bit of butter and seasoned with salt and pepper	Feta cheese and olives	Smoked salmon with cucumber and cream cheese: spread the cream cheese on the smoked salmon, add slices of cucumber and season with black pepper.

Thursday	Friday	Saturday	Sunday
Moussaka (page 98) with green salad (page 198)	Cream of spinach soup (page 79) with super seeded crackers (page 230)	One-pan prawn and chorizo skillet (page 114) A few squares of 85% or 90% dark chocolate – about the size of a credit card – with a couple of teaspoons of a nut butter spread on top	Red, amber, green frittata (page 50)
Stuffed red peppers (page 150) Greek yoghurt with frozen fruit (such as cherries or strawberries). This is really good if you defrost the fruit in the fridge for an hour or two before use.	Butter chicken (page 88) with cauliflower rice (page 216)	Eggs Florentine (page 44)	Pulled pork lettuce wraps (page 166) Chocolate mousse (page 195)
Ham/turkey, Cheddar and tomato roll-ups: place the cheese on top of the ham or turkey and top with sliced tomato. Season with salt and pepper and roll up.	Apple with 2 teaspoons of peanut butter	Hummus and cucumber	Handful of nuts such as walnuts or almonds with some Cheddar cheese

Sample Meal Planner 2

	Monday	Tuesday	Wednesday
First meal of the day – the time that you open your Eating Window	Prawn fishcakes (page 113) with carrot and poppy seed crunch (page 223)	Crab salad (page 64) A bowl of frozen berries topped with double cream	Roast red pepper and tomato soup (page 77)
Second meal	Soft-boiled eggs with asparagus soldiers (page 40)	Tofu schnitzel (page 92) with roast Brussels sprouts (page 221)	Pesto chicken and veg one-pan roast (page 85) Greek yoghurt topped with grated 85% or 90% dark chocolate and chopped hazelnuts
Snack	Cherry tomatoes (or a sliced regular tomato) with cheese	Celery sticks with peanut butter	Tin of tuna mashed up with mayonnaise and seasoned with salt and pepper

in full colou

Thursday	Friday	Saturday	Sunday
Herb and garlic lamb chops (page 97) with green dream broccoli mash (page 218)	Salmon rainbow parcels (page 117) with roasted broccoli with chilli, almonds and pecorino (page 204)	Marinated baked feta (page 206) with G3 salad (page 199) A few squares of 85% or 90% dark chocolate — about the size of a credit card — with a couple of teaspoons of clotted cream on top	Green eggs (page 47)
Full avo-salsa burrito (page 36)	Cauliflower crust pizza (page 134)	Steak and piri-piri slaw (page 101)	Classic roast chicken with sausage and sage stuffing (page 156) and steamed greens No-bake summer berry cheesecake (page 191)
Bowl of Greek yoghurt with blueberries	Apple and a handful of nuts	Vegetable crudités dipped in tzatziki	Avocado (half or whole depending on how strong your hunger signal is), cut in half, stone removed, either eaten as is or drizzled with tangy salad dressing (page 232)

Quick reference lists — what's the right recipe for right now?

You'll have noticed that at the top of every recipe, there's information on things like whether a recipe is a great portable option or if it's ideal for batch cooking. To help you to decide which recipes will suit you best at any particular time, I have summarized these recipe features in six easy-to-reference lists. Most recipes feature in more than one list, so you can choose from a list and then cross-reference to see if it also meets other criteria for the day's cooking, like it's ready in under 15 and it's vegan or there's a vegetarian option and it freezes well. I hope these lists prove helpful for selecting recipes that perfectly fit what you want to eat, when you want to eat it:

Ready in under 15

Eggs, salads and soups
- Omelette, p.52
- Fully loaded avocados, p.53
- Mozzarella, tomato and basil salad, p.55
- Sardine and roast pepper salad, p.68

Meat, fish and big veg
- Spiced tofu scramble, p.129
- Courgetti carbonara, p.151

Sides
- Green salad, p.198
- G3 salad, p.199
- Cauliflower rice, p.216

Essentials and drinks
- Tangy salad dressing, p.232
- Creamy salad dressing, p.233
- Mayonnaise, p.234
- Grapefruit and soda quencher, p.240

♈ Vegetarian or vegetarian option

Eggs, salads and soups
- Full avo-salsa burrito, p.36
- Avocado and black bean baked eggs, p.39
- Eggs Florentine, p.44
- Green eggs, p.47
- Omelette, p.52
- Fully loaded avocados, p.53
- Mozzarella, tomato and basil salad, p.55
- Burrata with tomato and summer veg salad, p.56
- Halloumi and caper salad, p.59
- The full house salad, p.60
- The full Caesar, p.63
- Falafel salad, p.74
- Chilled avocado soup, p.76
- Roast red pepper and tomato soup, p.77
- Cream of spinach soup, p.79
- Roast chickpea and cauliflower soup, p.80

in full colou

Great portable option

Ideal for batch cooking

❄ Freezes well

Celebration! menu inspiration

One of the most rewarding parts of running the Programme is when my patients report back how their Full Diet eating is their ticket to taking part in things again. From weddings to birthdays to special celebrations like Christmas, Diwali, Eid and Passover, food is no longer something to be feared, but instead it forms part of the richness of life and gathering together. In addition to my suggestions for Christmas (pages 154–5), I have written three sample Celebration menus for inspiration. Do use any elements of these for your own special occasions. You can also choose other ideas from the book as well as any recipes that you feel speak of happy times around a full table:

Celebration! Menu Inspiration 1

Pre-meal: Grapefruit and soda quencher (page 240) served with crunchy kale crisps (page 226) and a bowl of mixed olives

Starter: Burrata with tomato and summer veg salad (page 56)

Main: Whole lemon and herb-stuffed roast salmon with hollandaise (page 173) with green salad (page 198)

Pudding: Key lime pie (page 192)

Celebration! Menu Inspiration 2

Pre-meal: Cool cucumber and basil infusion (page 240) served with roasted almonds

Starter: Twice-baked cheese soufflé (page 182) with rocket

Main: Porchetta (page 162) with apple sauce (page 235), cauliflower cheese wedges (page 215) and steamed green beans

Pudding: Celebration watermelon layer cake (page 188)

Making every bit count

Putting ingredients in the bin which could otherwise be put to good use feels uncomfortable. Not only are we all now aware of the environmental impact of the food that we eat, but in the current climate in which food is increasingly expensive, I often talk with my patients at our Programme meetings about how we can use every last bit of an ingredient. Here are some of the suggestions that we've come up with:

Leftover chicken

Crispy skin:

This recipe makes use of any leftover cooked skin. Preheat the oven to 200°C/180°C fan/gas 6. Pat the chicken skins dry with kitchen paper. Place the skins on a baking sheet lined with baking parchment and season with sea salt. Cover with more baking parchment and place another baking tray on top to weigh the skins down. Bake for 10–15 minutes, until the skins are crisped up and golden. Remove and serve immediately.

Broth or stock:

This recipe is for about 1kg of bones. Adjust the recipe quantities according to the amount of bones you have.

Place the bones or roast carcass in a large saucepan along with a peeled, chopped carrot, 1 onion peeled and cut into quarters, a chopped stick of celery, 1 bashed unpeeled garlic clove, a chopped leek and fresh herbs tied in a bouquet garni, for example 2 sprigs of thyme, a bay leaf and 3 sprigs of parsley. Add 4 peppercorns and a clove. Cover with 2 litres of cold water and bring to the boil, then reduce the heat right down and simmer for 3 hours, skimming off any scum from the top when you need to. Pour through a sieve to remove the solid ingredients. Eat as a chicken broth or use for stock. Keeps in the fridge for 2 days. Alternatively, allow to cool and freeze for future use.

Salads or traybakes:

You can use leftover cooked chicken meat to make a salad (such as the full Caesar on page 63), it can be mashed up with mayonnaise, salt and pepper to make a chicken mayo or added to a vegetable traybake (like the one on page 138) 10 minutes before the end of the cooking time to warm the chicken through.

Leftover lemons and limes

For a delicious lime- or lemonade add the used juiced fruit to a jug of sparkling water and chill in the fridge. Alternatively store in the fridge and add a slice of leftover lemon or lime to hot water for a refreshing, caffeine-free drink. You can also chop the fruit up into wedges and freeze. Then add to water for a citrusy ice cube effect.

Leftover fresh herbs

If you have leftover fresh herbs, remove the stems, chop up the leaves and place in an ice cube tray. Cover with a dash of olive oil, fill the cube-mould with water, and freeze. When needed, you can tip the herb cube directly into your cooking if a little extra water won't disrupt things – as the cube melts, the herbs will infuse your dish. Alternatively, pop the frozen herb cube out, place in a bowl and, when melted, remove the herbs from the water and pat dry before using.

Leftover vegetables

Preheat the oven to 200°C/180°C fan/gas 6. Throw the leftover veg into a roasting tray, add a glug of olive oil and season with salt and pepper. You can also add some mixed herbs or, for a more smoky dish, some paprika, or anything else you like the taste of. Stir to coat the vegetables and roast for about 35–45 minutes (depending on which vegetables you are using). Alternatively, use the leftover veg in the chicken stock recipe (minus the chicken bones) to make a vegetable broth or stock.

Leftover egg yolks and whites

Beat a whole egg in with the leftover yolks or whites and use to make a scrambled egg or an omelette.

Five things I have learned about food (and everything else)

Running the Programme is a privilege. To meet people at the start, when they are often at their lowest ebb, and to share in their success as they lose weight, reinvigorate their health and start to live life to the full is a joy.

Over the years, I have changed too. I don't think it's possible to travel with people whose lives are changing before your eyes and not to reflect and learn yourself.

Within our group, I am there as the expert that shares the science, but I am not the only teacher in the room. Every group I meet either teaches me something new or reaffirms a thought that had been slowly taking flight, until finally it becomes an idea with wings.

This is what the Programme and my patients have taught me:

1. Food: Before I started the Programme, I was a competent cook. Talking food with my patients week after week, and learning from their knowledge and experience, has immeasurably elevated and enriched my own cooking. Here are the little bits of kitchen wisdom, shared by my patients, that have made all the difference:

i. Try to avoid cooking meat cold from the fridge. Taking it out of the fridge and allowing the temperature to come up a bit before cooking loosens up the meat fibres, which will change the whole eating experience.

ii. Cheese is also better if taken out of the fridge before use and allowed to warm up a bit first, which relaxes its natural creaminess and makes it even more delicious.

iii. To keep their sweet, umami flavour, store tomatoes out of the fridge.

iv. Nuts and seeds taste incredibly rich and flavoursome when roasted to bring out their natural oils. Tip on to a baking tray at 170°C/150°C fan/gas 3 and roast for about 10–15 minutes, shaking the tray regularly.

v. Boiling tap water and then pouring it into a bottle or jug and allowing it to cool, completely changes the taste because the boiling evaporates off the chlorine.

2. Don't let the perfect be the enemy of the good: Sometimes your Programme choices might not be as perfect as you would like. For example, you might only be able to go for a 20-minute walk rather than your usual hour. It's still worth getting that movement in because that 20 minutes will certainly benefit your physical health and be a welcome dose of mind first aid. Or you may find that an 8-hour Eating Window isn't practical for your own particular lifestyle or situation. In this case, it's still better to have a Window and to have it open for slightly longer, than not to have an Eating Window at all. The Programme has been designed in a real life setting. And sometimes life isn't perfect. Just do the best you can at that particular moment and be kind to yourself — don't let the perfect be the enemy of the good.

3. Sometimes showing up is enough: There are times when stuff doesn't work out. Taking a detour or stumbling along the way happens to all of us, whatever it

in full colour

is we are trying to achieve. When this happens in the Programme, time and again, I have been awed and inspired by my patients' tenacity and courage. When they could just miss a session because they were eating off-Programme or their weight loss had stalled, they have instead shown up. And at that particular point in their journey that was enough.

4. We are all a work in progress: Whether you are trying to get more sleep, quit ultra-processed food or move more during the day, these new behaviours will take time to become a natural part of your routine. When you do achieve these goals, they will still subtly and wonderfully change and grow the more you use them and the better they make you feel. In this way, whatever we want out of life, from weight loss to adapting our approach to parenting, learning a new language or getting even better at our job, we are all a work in progress. Rather than feeling any sense of weariness at this idea, instead I, and so many of my patients, find this a deeply encouraging and optimistic prospect.

5. Cooking can be the drumbeat of life: I hope you find, as many of my patients do, that your Full Diet cooking is not simply a daily routine, but instead takes on the dependable and steadfast rhythm of the drumbeat to a life that is moving forward. Like my patients, you too can develop a confidence and pride in creating meals that nourish you and your loved ones. You can view every dish, plate and bowl you prepare as a small act of love and self-care. As you cook, you will develop a quiet know-how that comes with fully tasting food again – a little bit more seasoning here, gentle with the fresh herbs there. Day after day you too can create food that becomes part of your own story in a way that mass-produced, made-for-profit food never could – the twice-baked soufflé at a milestone birthday, the day-trip bean salad eaten in the car to shelter from the rain. This book is a celebration of years of our Programme food and cooking. Of losing weight and gaining health. Of looking up at the stars with the confidence that your dreams and goals are possible. Of showing up and taking part. Of living life to the full.

acknowledgements

It is the clinical expertise, academic brilliance and kindness of my friends and colleagues at the Imperial Weight Centre that make being part of our Unit such a privilege. The support, encouragement and collaboration of these outstanding clinicians and scientists has given The Full Diet – or Imperial-SatPro – its wings. Amongst all of the pioneering, specialist work at the Imperial Weight Centre, the Programme has found its natural home and continues to evolve, flourish and change our patients' lives.

I am conscious of how lucky I am to know, learn from and work with Consultant Endocrinologists: Dr Harvey Chahal, Dr Chioma Izzi-Engbeaya, Dr Alex Miras and Professor Tricia Tan; Consultant Surgeons: Mr Ahmed Ahmed, Mr Sherif Hakky, Mr Krishna Moorthy, Ms Patricia Ortega, Mr Sanjay Purkayastha and Mr Christos Tsironis; Consultant Anaesthetist and Clinical Service Lead: Dr Jonathan Cousins; Consultant Anaesthetist: Dr Mark Catolico; Consultant Gastroenterologist: Dr Devinder Bansi; Consultant Psychiatrist: Dr Samantha Scholtz; Clinical Research Fellows: Dr Julia Kenkre and Dr Saleem Ansari; Diabetes Nurse Specialist: Anna Sackey; Clinical Nurse Specialists: Karen O'Donnell, Louisa Brolly and Ciara Price; and Specialist Dieticians: Candace Bovill-Taylor, Jo Boyle, Tamsin Hill, Rhian Houghton, Kate Parry and Jess Upton. Our clinical work is only possible because of our brilliant MDT co-ordinators: Debbie O'Rourke and Sahra Jama; the superb administrative support of Cathy Dolan and Khadra Hassan; and the highly effective management of Izabela Dubas and Anna Kennedy.

I am also incredibly fortunate to work at the Imperial Centre for Endocrinology under the exceptional leadership of Professor Karim Meeran. I am so very grateful to Prof for his mentorship, kindness and his unerring optimism – a meeting with Prof makes everything feel possible – including his suggestion to write Imperial Sat-Pro the book.

It was my scientific and academic training in the laboratory of Professor Sir Steve Bloom and Professor Waljit Dhillo at Imperial College London that gave me the skills, know-how and confidence to design the Programme. The greatest thanks are due to both Steve and Waljit for their wise guidance, supervision and support.

Very special thanks go to Professor Tricia Tan who from the outset immediately recognized the potential of the Programme and who has supported I-SatPro every step of the way. I am so grateful to Tricia for her kindness and encouragement and for all of her brilliant clinical and scientific contributions to the Programme which have been so greatly important to its success. I also thank the National Institute for Health and Care Research (NIHR) and the Imperial BRC for their funding support which made the original I-SatPro research study possible.

I owe immense gratitude to Dr Haya Alessimii who has been such an integral part of the Programme's story – from her superb work at the Clinical Research Facility to the compassionate care that she has brought to so many of our patient groups.

I thank my lucky stars that I get to work with my great friend Dr Vicky Salem who is academically and clinically brilliant and whose loyalty and exceptional kindness are ever sure and always give me courage.

In my fascinating conversations with Dr Boon Lim I have learnt so much about life as well as generous, intelligent, holistic patient care – I am very lucky to call Boon a friend. I am very grateful to James Harwood at London Metabolic Laboratory for his numerous clever ideas as an outstanding Programme coach and many, many thanks also to Sach Dunn and Vanessa Craig for their excellent PA support. Great thanks also to Mr Sanjay Purkayastha for his time, his kindness and superb advice on clinical matters and everything else.

I am deeply fortunate to be represented by my literary agent Will Francis. I owe huge gratitude to Will for the superb quality of his advice, his kindness and constant support. My first book, *The Full Diet*, and now this book would not exist without Will's exceptionally astute navigation and his enthusiasm from our first conversation for the idea of writing the Programme as a book. So many thanks also go to Will's highly effective, excellent colleagues at Janklow & Nesbit.

My brilliant publisher Fenella Bates at Penguin Michael Joseph is a joy to work with. I am new to the literary world, still I feel certain that finding that 'click' with somebody who has the remarkable combination of vision, creativity, commercial expertise and kindness must be a rare find. I owe the greatest thanks to Fenella for believing in me and for her utmost skill for turning good ideas into beautiful, tangible books. My editor Paula Flanagan does so much that to thank Paula solely for her editorial brilliance is not enough, this book and *The Full Diet* have been immeasurably enriched by Paula's diligence, incisive comments, meticulous organization and always knowing the answer to my many questions. Thank you also to Annie Lee for being such a thorough and smart copy-editor. I am also phenomenally grateful to Gaby Young, Jen Harlow, Ali Nazari and Vicky Photiou – the brilliant Penguin Michael Joseph publicity and marketing team – who have all worked so hard to share the Programme with thousands of readers beyond my Imperial NHS clinic.

As somebody who believes that the answer to most things can almost always be found in a book, I am totally thrilled that this book is not only practical but also looks so beautiful, for which so many thanks go to: Hannah Taylor-Eddington for her artful and brilliantly composed photographs, Sam Duff, Maria Gurevich and Jessica McIntosh, and Jake Fenton for making everything look both delicious and incredibly stylish, and Emma Leon whose kindness shines through in her work. The greatest thanks also go to Kat Mead. Kat's deep knowledge, expertise and hard work have been absolutely instrumental in professionalizing, polishing and perfecting the ideas of a home cook into a collection of beautiful and deliciously good recipes.

I am also very grateful to the innovative and imaginative Penguin Michael Joseph design team, Daniel Prescott-Bennett and Sarah Fraser, who have used their great skill and creativity to beautifully draw the book together.

It's pretty lucky when writing a cookbook to have Michael Greenwold's number on speed dial. Very many thanks go to Michael for his sparkling advice on the manuscript and – as far back as the days when I was taller than him – for teaching me so much about food and cooking

I am so very grateful to my best friend Lauren Mishcon for almost forty years of love, unwavering support and on-going conversation, who so generously read and gave greatly appreciated feedback on the recipes. Life is immeasurably enriched by the love, constancy and camaraderie of my oldest and dearest friends who are also my family: Misha Moore, Vicky Salem, Mark Nichols, Elizabeth Lands, Fariha Sultan and Farima and Duncan Perry. Great thanks and much gratitude also go to Simona Vasile and Veronica Casian whose help, care and kindness over so many years is a gift we treasure.

Now that I am a mother I can see anew how extraordinary my mum Christine Hameed is in her energy, loyalty, support and the great interest she has in all of us — always nurturing and caring about the things that her children consider important. This book is dedicated to my dazzling dad, Dr Khalid Hameed, around whose table everyone gathers for his delicious and always abundant food — but more than that — being at the table together is a blessing because of the generous, great and brilliant man sitting at the head. I am forever thankful for the love, friendship and comfort of my three magnificent siblings Hasan, Imran and Amna Hameed whose company always feels like coming home. I am very fortunate to be part of such a large family and the love and care that binds us all including: Ghazala Hameed, Sophia Javaid Hameed, Asad Khan, Reza Javaid, Alia Brahimi, Noor and Lara Hameed, Spencer Eade, Max, Natalie, Stella and Clara Eade and Michael and Tara Greenwold. There's a saying that — when you marry the boy, you marry the family — which is fantastically lucky for me because the love, care and support that Lynn and Steve Greenwold have shown me ever since I was a medical student has been extraordinary in its generosity, depth and impact.

This book exists because of the love and dedication of my husband Jonathan Greenwold and the unending belief that he has in me. Jonathan's love, care, energy, attention and generosity is extraordinary and is the foundation on which my world is built — my home is wherever Jonathan is. Our lives are so full and bright because of Sibella, Teddy, Hal and Raphael Bear — who constantly amaze and inspire me with their intelligence, curiosity and sheer love of life — my heart is full with wonderful you.

And lastly the greatest thanks are for my patients whose courage, determination and generosity run through the heart of the Programme. Thank you for inviting me to share your inspirational journey over so many years; it is a privilege to know you and to be part of your beautiful story.

index

index

notes